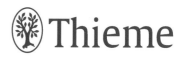

Neuroradiology Q&A for the Radiology Boards

Michael Iv, MD
Clinical Associate Professor of Radiology (Neuroradiology)
Stanford University Medical Center
Stanford, California, USA

228 illustrations

Thieme
New York • Stuttgart • Delhi • Rio de Janeiro

Library of Congress Cataloging-in-Publication Data
is available from the publisher.

Important note: Medicine is an ever-changing science undergoing continual development. Research and clinical experience are continually expanding our knowledge, in particular our knowledge of proper treatment and drug therapy. Insofar as this book mentions any dosage or application, readers may rest assured that the authors, editors, and publishers have made every effort to ensure that such references are in accordance with **the state of knowledge at the time of production of the book.**

Nevertheless, this does not involve, imply, or express any guarantee or responsibility on the part of the publishers in respect to any dosage instructions and forms of applications stated in the book. **Every user is requested to examine carefully** the manufacturers' leaflets accompanying each drug and to check, if necessary in consultation with a physician or specialist, whether the dosage schedules mentioned therein or the contraindications stated by the manufacturers differ from the statements made in the present book. Such examination is particularly important with drugs that are either rarely used or have been newly released on the market. Every dosage schedule or every form of application used is entirely at the user's own risk and responsibility. The authors and publishers request every user to report to the publishers any discrepancies or inaccuracies noticed. If errors in this work are found after publication, errata will be posted at www.thieme.com on the product description page.

Some of the product names, patents, and registered designs referred to in this book are in fact registered trademarks or proprietary names even though specific reference to this fact is not always made in the text. Therefore, the appearance of a name without designation as proprietary is not to be construed as a representation by the publisher that it is in the public domain.

Thieme addresses people of all gender identities equally. We encourage our authors to use gender-neutral or gender-equal expressions wherever the context allows.

Thieme Medical Publishers, Inc.
333 Seventh Avenue, 18th Floor,
New York, NY 10001, USA
www.thieme.com
+1 800 782 3488, customerservice@thieme.com

Cover design: © Thieme
Cover image source: © PIC4U/stock.adobe.com
Typesetting by Thomson Digital, India

Printed in Germany by Beltz Grafische Betriebe

5 4 3 2 1

ISBN 978-1-68420-559-2

Also available as an e-book:
eISBN (PDF): 978-1-68420-125-9
eISBN (epub): 978-1-68420-560-8

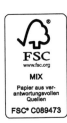

I dedicate this book to my husband, Robert, whose unwavering support, understanding, and patience have allowed me to realize my hopes, dreams, and ambitions.

Contents

Contents

Preface

For many residents, fellows, and practicing radiologists, preparation for the Core, Certifying, and/or Subspecialty ABR Exams involves several months (if not years) of reading text, interpretating images, and answering questions. Sitting for one of these exams, which were developed to test one's knowledge and understanding of anatomy, pathophysiology, and physics concepts that are important in diagnostic imaging, represents a stressful yet crucial time in a radiologist's life, as board certification is an essential component to practice medicine. With regards to neuroradiology, these image-rich exams span the breadth of brain, spine, and head and neck imaging. As such, the primary motivation for writing this book is to help prepare for and ace these exams. Outside of the exam setting, it may also be useful as a refresher for those looking to brush up on their clinical neuroimaging skills.

This book consists of a collection of 100 "standard difficulty" and "challenging" cases, each selected to illustrate specific pathology and draw out teaching points that one might (and likely will) encounter in exams and in the reading room. Each case begins with two or three high-quality images, followed by three questions that assess comprehension of imaging diagnosis, histopathology, and management. To cover potentially testable material, cases were selected from all areas of neuroradiology and include pathology in adults and children. A group of bright, young, academic neuroradiologists at Stanford University who recently took the Core and Certifying Exams (and who went through the same journey of studying and answering endless, multiple-choice questions on computers) contributed to the compilation of cases and writing of questions.

All of us involved in assembling this book are passionate about teaching and education and want to play our part in helping current and future generations of radiologists improve their clinical skills, which will ultimately improve patient care. In the end, paying it forward is what it is truly about!

Michael Iv, MD

Acknowledgment

I would like to acknowledge all the contributors to this book. I appreciate their time and dedication to enhance radiology education and truly hope that they see the fruits of their labor. Each contributor is a junior faculty member, colleague, and friend, who makes my work enjoyable and meaningful. To infinity and beyond!

Contributors

Syed Hashmi, MD
Clinical Assistant Professor of Radiology
(Neuroradiology)
Stanford University
Stanford, California, USA

Bryan Lanzman, MD
Clinical Assistant Professor of Radiology
(Neuroradiology)
Stanford University
Stanford, California, USA

Mrudula Penta, MD
Clinical Assistant Professor of Radiology
(Neuroradiology)
Stanford University
Stanford, California, USA

Eric Tranvinh, MD
Clinical Assistant Professor of Radiology
(Neuroradiology)
Stanford University
Stanford, California, USA

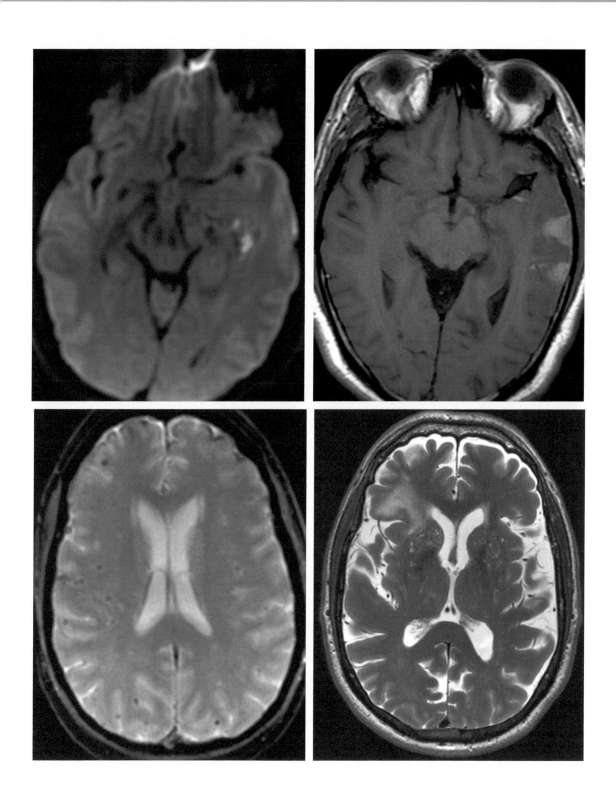

Please refer to the following images to answer the next three questions:

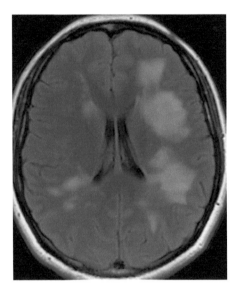 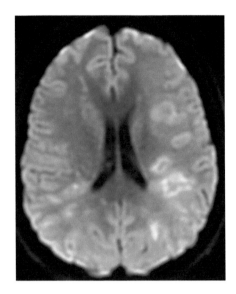

A 24-year-old female with recent influenza immunization presents with headaches, difficulty in speaking, and weakness of the left arm and leg.

1.1 What is the **MOST** likely diagnosis given the patient's history and imaging findings?

A. Multiple sclerosis.
B. Acute disseminated encephalomyelitis.
C. Metastatic disease.
D. Viral encephalitis.
E. Septic emboli.

1.2 Which of the following **BEST** characterizes the natural history of ADEM as seen in the majority of patients?

A. Monophasic, self-limited.
B. Rapidly progressive.
C. Relapsing–remitting.
D. Biphasic.
E. Multiphasic.

1.3 With regard to ADEM, which of the following is **TRUE**?

A. Normal brain magnetic resonance imaging (MRI) excludes the diagnosis of ADEM.
B. Elevated oligoclonal bands are frequently found in cerebrospinal fluid (CSF) studies.
C. Deep gray matter involvement is more typical of multiple sclerosis (MS) than of ADEM.
D. Bilateral optic neuritis is a common presenting sign.
E. Treatment includes whole brain radiation and chemotherapy.

Answers and Explanations

1.1 Correct: B. Acute disseminated encephalomyelitis.

Peripheral (often incomplete) rings of restricted diffusion and enhancement (not shown) associated with T2/fluid-attenuated inversion recovery (FLAIR) hyperintense white matter lesions are characteristic of acute disseminated encephalomyelitis (ADEM). The presence of restricted diffusion and enhancement, which are typically, but not always, present in ADEM, indicates acute disease and active demyelination. This is true across many of the demyelinating diseases, so these features cannot be used to distinguish between the different disease types of demyelinating diseases. Clinical history and laboratory correlation is therefore necessary. ADEM is characterized by acute autoimmune-mediated inflammation and demyelination of the white matter (and to a lesser extent gray matter) of the brain and spinal cord, typically occurring within days to weeks after infection or vaccination. Lesions are usually bilateral and asymmetric, and may or may not involve the thalami and brainstem. This condition usually occurs in children or adolescents, although it can occur at any age.

Other choices and discussion

A. The imaging findings of multiple sclerosis (MS) can and often do overlap with those of ADEM, but there are key differences in the clinical history. Specifically, MS is often a chronic and progressive disease that is characterized by lesions that are disseminated in space (i.e., different parts of the brain and spinal cord) and time, while ADEM is typically self-limited and monophasic. Also, MS tends to occur in patients who are older than those with ADEM. Characteristic white matter lesions of MS are those that are periventricular in location, oriented perpendicularly relative to the plane of the lateral ventricles ("Dawson's fingers"), and involve the callososeptal interface. In contrast, the corpus callosum is usually not involved in ADEM.
C. Parenchymal metastatic disease often occurs at the gray–white matter junction and is not usually isolated to the white matter as in the above case. In addition, the absence of a known history of primary malignancy makes this diagnosis unlikely.
D. Multifocal pyogenic microabscesses classically exhibit central restricted diffusion on diffusion-weighted imaging. The white matter lesions in this case have a peripheral and incomplete ring of diffusion restriction, an imaging feature that is characteristic of demyelinating disease.
E. As with other hematogenous processes, septic emboli often occurs at the corticomedullary junction and is not typically confined to the white matter as in the case above. In many cases, the lesions are predominantly found in a vascular distribution and frequently associated with ischemia and/or hemorrhage.

1.2 Correct: A. Monophasic, self-limited.

Acute disseminated encephalomyelitis (ADEM) is usually monophasic and self-limited with complete recovery occurring within one to six months, which is seen in 50 to 70% of cases. Neurologic sequelae (especially those presenting with optic neuropathy) are seen in 10 to 20% of patients. Poorer prognosis is associated with multiple factors including unresponsiveness to steroids, severe neurological symptoms, and attacks without accompanying fevers. Children also tend to have more favorable outcomes than adults.

Other choices and discussion

B. A rapidly progressive form of ADEM—acute hemorrhagic encephalomyelitis or leukoencephalitis—occurs in approximately 2% of patients with ADEM. This variant form is characterized by hemorrhage and necrosis of vessel walls, and usually occurs in young patients with abrupt and severe symptom onset. In addition, there exists an association with ulcerative colitis and asthma. While ADEM is classically monophasic, several large pediatric studies have shown that relapses do occur, but with variable frequency.
C. According to the International Pediatric multiple sclerosis (MS) Study Group, relapsing–remitting disease occurrence beyond a second attack often indicates a chronic disorder, most often leading to the diagnosis of MS or neuromyelitis optica.
D. Biphasic disseminated encephalomyelitis is not included in the current consensus guidelines from the International Pediatric MS Study Group.
E. According to the International Pediatric MS Study Group, multiphasic disseminated encephalomyelitis is defined as experiencing a second attack separated by 3 months but not followed by any further events. The second attack can involve either a new anatomic area or a reemergence of prior neurologic symptoms or signs of disease. There is a much lower observed frequency of a multiphasic than a monophasic disease.

1.3 Correct: D. Bilateral optic neuritis is a common presenting sign.

Bilateral optic neuritis is a common presenting sign of ADEM. In contrast, unilateral optic neuropathy occurs much more frequently in patients with MS. Among patients with ADEM, those presenting with optic neuropathy often have persistent or chronic symptoms even after resolution of the initial clinical episode.

Other choices and discussion

A. The statement that a normal brain MRI excludes the diagnosis of ADEM is false. While lesions of ADEM often appear simultaneously with the clinical presentation and resolve with clinical recovery, there is sometimes a delay (up to 1 month) between symptom onset and MRI abnormalities. Therefore, a normal brain MRI does not exclude the diagnosis of ADEM, and follow-up is recommended if there is strong clinical evidence for this diagnosis.

B. Elevated oligoclonal bands in CSF are rare and typically transient, but can occur in approximately 12.5% of pediatric patients with ADEM. In contrast, oligoclonal bands in the CSF are present in at least 80% of MS cases.

C. The statement that deep gray matter involvement is more typical of MS than of ADEM is false. In fact, the opposite is true: deep gray matter (e.g., thalami or basal ganglia) involvement is more characteristic of ADEM than of MS. Also, the cerebral cortex is involved in approximately 30% of ADEM cases. Aggressive treatment targeted at rapidly reducing inflammation is the goal of therapy for ADEM. The early use of high-dose steroids, which is a widely accepted first-line treatment, contributes to an improved prognosis. In the majority of cases, lesions resolve completely with corticosteroid therapy. Additional immunosuppressive therapies such as intravenous immunoglobulin, cyclophosphamide, and plasmaphresis have also been shown to be beneficial.

E. Whole brain radiation and chemotherapy are treatments for neoplastic disease involving the central nervous system, not ADEM.

References

Krupp LB, Banwell B, Tenembaum S, for the International Pediatric MS Study Group. Consensus definitions proposed for pediatric multiple sclerosis and related disorders. *Neurology*. 2007; 68(Suppl 2):S7–S12.

Krupp LB, Tardieu M, Amato MP, for the International Pediatric MS Study Group. International Pediatric Multiple Sclerosis Group criteria for pediatric multiple sclerosis and immune-mediated central nervous system demyelinating disorders: revisions to the 2007 definitions. *Mult Scler*. 2013;19:1261–1267.

Menge T, Kieseier BC, Nessler S, et al. Acute disseminated encephalomyelitis: an acute hit against the brain. *Curr Opin Neurol*. 2007;20:247–254.

Rossi A. Imaging of acute disseminated encephalomyelitis. *Neuroimag Clin N Am*. 2008;18:149–161.

Please refer to the following images to answer the next three questions:

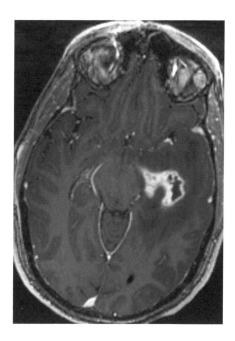
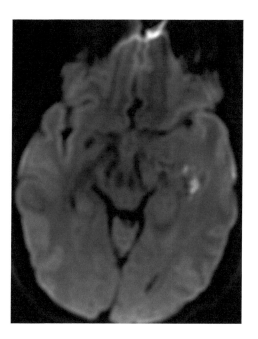

A 41-year-old male from Central Valley, California, presents with fever and new onset seizure.

2.1 Which of the following imaging feature is **MOST** specific for a cerebral abscess?

A. Restricted diffusion within the lesion core.

B. Peripheral or rim enhancement.

C. T2/fluid-attenuated inversion recovery (FLAIR) signal surrounding the lesion.

D. Mass effect on surrounding structures.

E. Hypointense gradient echo (GRE) signal within the lesion core.

2.2 Given the patient's history and imaging findings, including marked basilar leptomeningeal enhancement (not shown), which of the following is the **MOST** likely responsible organism?

A. *Coccidioides immitis.*

B. *Cryptococcus neoformans.*

C. *Staphylococcus aureus.*

D. *Mycobacterium tuberculosis.*

E. *Treponema pallidum.*

2.3 Which of the following is typical of pyogenic or fungal abscesses on magnetic resonance spectroscopy?

A. Increased N-acetylaspartate (NAA) and creatine; decreased choline.

B. Decreased lipid and lactate.

C. Increased glutamine and glutamate.

D. Decreased cytosolic amino acids.

E. Increased cytosolic amino acids.

Answers and Explanations

2.1 Correct: A. Restricted diffusion within the lesion core.

Diffusion restriction with low apparent diffusion coefficient (ADC) values in the central cavity of pyogenic abscesses is virtually always present. Low ADC values can be seen with tubercular and fungal abscesses, although these tend to be more variable. The diffusion abnormality results from intact inflammatory cells in pus which impede the microscopic motion of water molecules. Restricted diffusion in intracavitary projections and the walls of fungal abscesses has also been demonstrated.

Other choices and discussion
B. While cerebral abscesses frquently show well-defined rim enhancement on postcontrast imaging (corresponding to an organized and formed capsule), peripheral or rim enhancement is seen in many other conditions such as metastases, primary brain tumors such as glioblastoma or lymphoma in immunocompromised patients, subacute infarcts, contusions, demyelinating diseases, and radiation necrosis.
C. The enhancement in abscesses is typically thin, smooth, and thinner along the medial margin. T2/FLAIR signal abnormality surrounding the lesion represents vasogenic edema and is a nonspecific finding that is present in many infectious, inflammatory, vascular, and malignant conditions.
D. Mass effect on surrounding structures is a nonspecific finding that is related to any space-occupying mass—the larger the mass, the greater the mass effect.
E. Hypointense GRE signal within the lesion core is not typical of cerebral pyogenic abscess. Instead, the rim or capsule of the cerebral abscess is typically iso-intense-to-hyperintense on T1-weighted images and hypointense on T2- and T2*(GRE)-weighted images.

2.2 Correct: A. *Coccidioides immitis.*

Coccidioides immitis is a fungus endemic to the soil of the southwestern United States, Mexico, and Central and South America, occurring most frequently among pregnant women, immunocompromised patients, and persons of Hispanic, Filipino, and African descent. Central nervous system involvement is the most frequent and severe manifestation of disseminated disease. Common brain imaging features include basilar meningitis, infarcts, periventricular white matter abnormalities, vasculitis, and parenchymal masses and abscesses.

Other choices and discussion
B. *Cryptococcus neoformans* is an opportunistic fungus best known for causing meningitis (often basilar meningitis) in immunosuppressed individuals, typically those afflicted with HIV/AIDS. It is found in the droppings of birds, often pigeons. Central nervous system (CNS) infection is related to hematogeneous dissemination from the lungs; once in the brain, the infection spreads along perivascular spaces to deep structures of the brain. Most pyogenic causes of meningitis are related to Streptococcus pneumonia, Neisseria meningitides, Group B streptococcus, Listeria monocytogenes, and Gram-negative bacilli, with the incidence of bacteria based on age.
C. *Staphyloccous aureus* meningitis is relatively uncommon and can be seen in association with neurosurgical intervention, congenital dermal sinus tract, or in the setting bacteremia from an extra-CNS source.
D. CNS infection due to *Mycobacterium tuberculosis* has many overlapping clinical and imaging features with CNS coccidioidomycosis. In the absence of a history of travel to an endemic country and HIV/AIDS, *Coccidioides immitis* is a better choice.
E. Neurosyphilis due to *Treponema pallidum* also has many overlapping clinical and imaging features with CNS coccidioidomycosis. Given the patient's history of fever and location, *Coccidioides immitis* is a better choice.

2.3 Correct: E. Increased cytosolic amino acids.

Increased cytosolic amino acid levels (0.9 ppm) are common in pyogenic and fungal abscesses due to the breakdown of neutrophils, subsequent release of proteolytic enzymes, and hydrolysis of proteins into amino acids.

Other choices and discussion
A. Increased NAA and creatine; decreased choline is incorrect. NAA (2.0 ppm) indicates neuronal integrity, creatine (3.0 ppm) indicates metabolism of energy, and choline (3.2 ppm) indicates membrane turnover. The opposite pattern, reduced NAA and creatine and elevated choline, is more consistent with an active metabolic process in the brain such as tumor or demyelination. Evaluating other metabolic peaks (amino acids, lipids, and lactates) is more helpful in diagnosing bacterial or fungal abscesses.
B. Decreased lipid and lactate is incorrect. The presence of lipid (1.2–1.3 ppm) and lactate (1.3 ppm) peaks are typical of pyogenic and fungal abscesses.
C. Increased glutamine and glutamate (represented by the Glx peak, 2.1–2.55 ppm) can be found in patients with hyperammonemia.
D. Conversely, decreased cytosolic amino acids is false. Succinate (2.4 ppm) and acetate (1.9 ppm) are also found in pyogenic and fungal abscesses, as these are end products of fermentation. Fungal abscesses, however, have multiple signal peaks between 3.6 and 3.8 ppm due to the presence of disaccharide trehalose.

References

Gupta NA, Iv M, Pandit RP, et al. Imaging manifestations of primary and disseminated coccidioidomycosis. *Applied Radiology*. 2015; 44:9–21.

Lammering JC, Iv M, Gupta N, et al. Imaging spectrum of CNS coccidioidomycosis: prevalence and significance of concurrent brain and spinal disease. *AJR Am J Roentgenol*. 2013; 200:1334–1346.

Luthra G, Parihar A, Nath K, et al. Comparative evaluation of fungal, tubercular, and pyogenic brain abscesses with conventional and diffusion MR imaging and proton MR spectroscopy. AJNR Am J Neuroradiol. 2007; 28:1332–1338.

Case 3

Please refer to the following images to answer the next three questions:

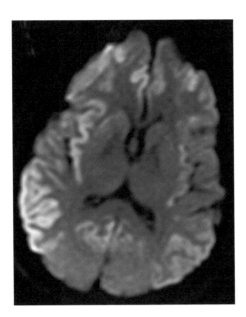

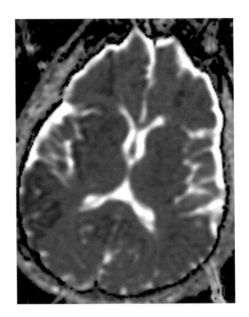

A 52-year-old female with rapidly progressive dementia and behavioral changes.

3.1 What is the **MOST** likely diagnosis, given the patient's history and negative early laboratory workup?

A. Hypoxic ischemic injury.

B. Creutzfeldt-Jakob disease (CJD).

C. Viral encephalitis.

D. Carbon monoxide poisoning.

E. Acute hyperammonemic encephalopathy.

3.2 Which of the following cortical areas is/are most frequently spared in sporadic Creutzfeldt-Jakob disease (CJD)?

A. Insula.

B. Cingulate gyrus.

C. Pre and postcentral gyri.

D. Precuneus.

E. Paracentral lobule.

3.3 With regard to Creutzfeldt-Jakob disease (CJD), which of the following is **TRUE**:

A. Typical electroencephalogram (EEG) findings are continuous high-voltage sharp waves.

B. Genetic CJD is caused by mutations in the prion protein gene (PRNP).

C. Sporadic CJD (sCJD) is also known as mad cow disease.

D. "Hockey stick sign" refers to signal abnormality of the caudate and putamen.

E. Definite diagnosis can be made by observing increased 14–3–3 protein in cerebrospinal fluid (CSF).

Answers and Explanations

3.1 Correct: B. Creutzfeldt-Jakob disease (CJD).

Four variants of CJD, a prion disease, have been described: sporadic CJD (sCJD, responsible for 85% of human prion diseases), genetic CJD (responsible for 10–15% of cases), and acquired CJD (iatrogenic CJD or variant CJD, which is responsible for fewer than 1% of cases). The clinical presentation is of a rapidly progressive dementia, with a constellation of pyramidal, extrapyramidal, and cerebellar signs, leading to death within less than one year. Classic imaging findings of CJD include progressive T2 hyperintensity and restricted diffusion involving the cerebral cortices, basal ganglia (especially caudate and putamen), and thalami (most common in variant CJD). Three cerebrospinal fluid (CSF) proteins (14–3–3 protein, total tau [τ-tau], and neuron-specific enolase [NSE]), have been used as biomarkers for CJD diagnosis, although these are usually only ordered when CJD is strongly suspected. Notably, magnetic resonance imaging (MRI) with diffusion-weighted imaging (DWI) has been reported to have a higher diagnostic accuracy than any or all of these three CSF protein biomarkers.

Other choices and discussion

A. Hypoxic ischemic injury does not present as a rapidly progressive dementia. Also, an inciting event (e.g., cardiac arrest, drowning, and asphyxiation) can usually be identified to explain the abnormal imaging findings. Hypoxic ischemic injury has variable imaging features depending on the severity of the hypoxic event. Restricted diffusion of the gray matter structures including the cerebral cortex, basal ganglia, thalami, hippocampi, and cerebellum is observed with severe hypoxic ischemic injury, whereas borderzone or watershed infarcts are seen with mild to moderate injury.

C. The clinical presentation of viral encephalitis is generally nonspecific and may include a variety of neurologic symptoms. Although rapid progressive dementia in the acute setting is a less frequent manifestation of viral infection (when compared to CJD), it can occur, particularly in younger patients. Viral encephalitides can involve any part of the brain (white matter, cortex, deep gray structures including the basal ganglia and thalami, brainstem, and cerebellum), with preferential involvement dependent on the specific organism. Involvement is manifested on imaging as T2/fluid-attenuated inversion recovery (FLAIR) hyperintensity with or without restricted diffusion. The imaging findings also overlap with CJD, and a combination of imaging and ancillary workup is necessary to ultimately determine the underlying etiology.

D. Carbon monoxide poisoning does not typically present as a rapidly progressive dementia. Patients can present with acute symptoms (nausea, vomiting, and headache) or chronic symptoms (cognitive decline, and gait disturbance). Definitive diagnosis lies in measuring the amount of carbon monoxide in the blood (carboxyhemoglobin). The typical finding of carbon monoxide poisoning on MRI is symmetric abnormal signal intensity in the globus pallidi on T1-weighted, T2-weighted, and DWI, which is absent in this case. In addition to necrosis and infarction of the globus pallidi, superimposed hemorrhage can occur.

E. Patients with acute hyperammonemic encephalopathy, commonly encountered in very sick patients being treated in the intensive care unit (ICU) and in patients with acute hepatic dysfunction, present with progressive drowsiness, seizures, and coma. Prolonged hyperammonemia can lead to long-term neurologic sequelae and significant brain injury. Acute hyperammonemic encephalopathy often demonstrates symmetric restricted diffusion of the cingulate gyri and insular cortices. Additional cortical involvement can be more variable and asymmetric.

3.2 Correct: C. Pre and postcentral gyri.

The precentral and postcentral gyri are spared approximately 60% and 70% of the time in sporadic CJD (sCJD), respectively.

Other choices and discussion

A and **B.** Cortical signal abnormalities in sCJD most frequently affect the insula and cingulate gyrus at a frequency of 95%.

D and **E.** The precuneus and paracentral lobule are affected in 85% and 77%, respectively.

3.3 Correct: B. Genetic CJD is caused by mutations in the prion protein gene (PRNP).

Ten to 15% of human prion disease cases are associated with mutations in the PRNP, which is located on chromosome 20. Prion protein is a normal host protein on the surface of many cells, particularly neurons. More than 30 PRNP mutations have been identified, leading to distinct clinicopathological syndromes.

Other choices and discussion

A. Typical EEG findings are periodic high-voltage sharp waves superimposed on a background of low-voltage activity, rather than continuous high-voltage sharp waves.

C. Sporadic CJD (sCJD) is the idiopathic form of CJD. Variant (vCJD) or new-variant CJD is known as mad cow disease or bovine spongiform encephalopathy and is related to ingestion of infected beef.

D. The "hockey stick sign" refers to T2/fluid-attenuated inversion recovery (FLAIR) hyperintense signal involving the dorsomedial thalamus and posterior thalamus (pulvinar), and not the caudate and putamen. It is seen in most cases of vCJD, but this sign can also be seen in other forms of CJD.

E. Identification of 14–3–3 protein in CSF makes the diagnosis of CJD probable but not definite. Definite diagnosis is made by brain biopsy or autopsy.

References

Caobelli F, Cobelli M, Pizzocaro C, et al. The role of neuroimaging in evaluating patients affected by Creutzfeldt-Jakob disease: a systematic review of the literature. *J Neuroimaging*. 2015; 25:2–13.

Grossman RI, Yousem DM, eds. Neuroradiology: The Requisites. Philadelphia, PA: Mosby, 2003.

Kim MO, Geschwind MD. Clinical update of Jakob-Creutzfeldt disease. *Curr Opin Neurol*. 2015;28: 302–310.

Tschampa HJ, Kallenberg K, Kretzschmar HA, et al. Pattern of cortical changes in sporadic Creutzfeldt-Jakob Disease. AJNR Am *J Neuroradiol*. 2007;28(6):1114–1118.

Case 4

Please refer to the following images to answer the next three questions:

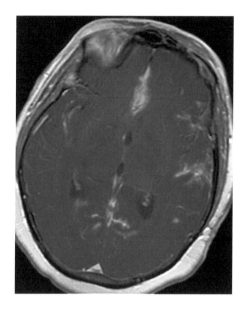 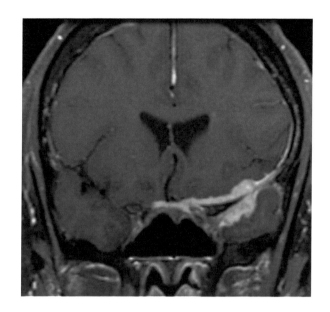

Two different patients with history withheld.

4.1 What is the **MOST** likely diagnosis, accounting for abnormal chest X-rays (not shown), in these patients?

A. Primary central nervous system (CNS) lymphoma.
B. Leptomeningeal carcinomatosis.
C. Bacterial meningitis.
D. Neurosarcoidosis.
E. En plaque meningioma.

4.2 Approximately what percentage of people with neurosarcoidosis have pulmonary involvement?

A. 1%.
B. 30%.
C. 50%.
D. 75%.
E. 90%.

4.3 What is the classic histologic hallmark of sarcoidosis?

A. Pseudopalisading necrosis.
B. Caseating granuloma.
C. Noncaseating granuloma.
D. Physaliphorous cell.
E. Small round blue cell.

Answers and Explanations

4.1 Correct: D. Neurosarcoidosis.

A wide spectrum of magnetic resonance (MR) manifestations of neurosarcoidosis exists and includes dural thickening and enhancement, leptomeningeal enhancement (most frequently affecting the suprasellar and frontal basal meninges), cranial nerve enhancement, enhancing extra-axial and parenchymal masses, lacunar infarcts, and pituitary stalk/hypothalamus thickening. Spine involvement is seen in 25% of cases. T2-hypointense lesions correlate to fibrocollagenous and gliotic tissue in dural lesions, whereas T2-hyperintense lesions correlate with inflammatory infiltrates. A high concentration of serum angiotensin-converting enzyme (ACE) is present in only 24 to 76% of cases and can be found in other conditions such as tuberculosis and malignancy, so it has limited diagnostic value. However, ACE levels are useful in diagnosing sarcoid involvement of the meninges and in monitoring disease course and treatment. Imaging findings in the cases above include pronounced and diffuse leptomeningeal enhancement involving the basilar cisterns and cerebral sulci and nodular dural enhancement along the floor of the left anterior cranial fossa and roof of the left middle cranial fossa.

Other choices and discussion

A. Meningeal enhancement is not typical for primary CNS lymphoma, arguing against this answer choice. Classic imaging findings of primary CNS lymphoma, which is most commonly a diffuse large B-cell, non-Hodgkin type, are enhancing lesion(s) that show restricted diffusion within the basal ganglia and periventricular white matter. There is also usually no other remote site of involvement.
B. Leptomeningeal carcinomatosis is a term for *subarachnoid* seeding of metastatic disease, occurring with many adult tumors such as glioblastoma, lymphoma, melanoma, and breast, lung, gastrointestinal, and genitourinary cancers. The second patient (right image) has dural involvement, so leptomeningeal carcinomatosis does not accurately describe the dural or pachymeningeal disease that is present.
C. Bacterial meningitis is often characterized by an abnormal leptomeningeal enhancement pattern rather than a pachymeningeal pattern as seen in the second patient (right image).
E. En plaque meningiomas are defined by a sheet-like appearance of dural involvement, which is often located in or near the sphenoid wing. While this may be on the differential for the second patient (right image), the first patient (left image) has leptomeningeal rather than dural-based enhancement. En plaque meningiomas comprise 2 to 9% of all meningiomas.

4.2 Correct: E. 90%.

Greater than 90% of patients with neurosarcoidosis have pulmonary involvement including bilateral hilar lymphadenopathy, diffuse lung infiltrations, and/or fibrosis depending on the stage of disease. These abnormalities are often identified on chest X-ray and/or computed tomography (CT).

Other choices and discussion

A–D. The other choices are incorrect. However, 1% of patients with neurosarcoidosis have disease isolated to the central nervous system (CNS), 30% of patients have skin involvement, and approximately 50% of patients have ocular involvement.

4.3 Correct: C. Noncaseating granuloma.

Noncaseating granuloma is found on hisopathology in about 80% of sarcoidosis cases. While noncaseating granulomas are characteristic of sarcoid, they are not absolutely specific for this disease as they can be found in a variety of other conditions.

Other choices and discussion

A. Pseudopalisading necrosis is a common feature of glioblastoma. Pseudopalisades are characterized by tumor cells surrounding a central clear zone. Small pseudopalisades may have internal fibrillary processes and apoptotic cells but lack central necrosis. Large pseudopalisades often contain regions of necrosis.
B. Caseating granuloma is a typical feature of tuberculosis and fungal infections. Caseating refers to the gross appearance of tissue necrosis, which is cheese-like in appearance.
D. Physaliphorous cells are large cells with vacuolated cytoplasms found in chordomas.
E. Small round blue cells are found within many tumors including primitive neuroectodermal tumors (e.g., medulloblastoma), retinoblastoma, and neuroblastoma. They are not a feature of sarcoidosis.

References

Kimura-Hayama ET, Higuera JA, Corona-Cedillo R, et al. Neurocysticercosis: radiologic-pathologic correlation. *Radiographics*. 2010;30(6):1705-1719.

Lucato LT, Guedes MS, Sato JR, et al. The role of conventional MR imaging sequences in the evaluation of neurocysticercosis: impact on characterization of the scolex and lesion burden. AJNR Am *J Neuroradiol*. 2007;28(8):1501–4.

Osborn AG. Parasitic Infections. In: Osborn AG, Hedlund GL, editors. Osborn's Brain: Imaging, Pathology, and Anatomy. 2nd ed. Philadelphia: Elsevier; 2018: 390–399.

Case 5

Please refer to the following images to answer the next three questions:

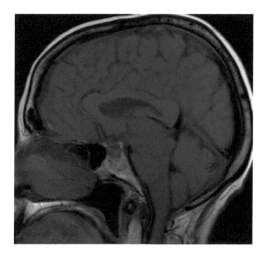 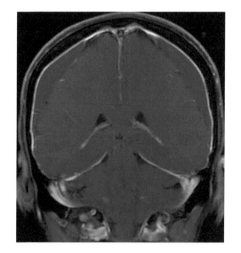

A 74-year-old female presents with severe headache.

5.1 Which is the **BEST** diagnosis for the above patient?

A. Bilateral subdural hematomas.

B. Hypertrophic pachymeningitis.

C. Chiari 1 malformation.

D. Intracranial hypotension.

E. Idiopathic intracranial hypertension.

5.2 Which of the following has been implicated as a cause for the underlying diagnosis?

A. Cranial cerebrospinal fluid (CSF) leak.

B. Brain tumor.

C. Disc-osteophyte.

D. Craniospinal irradiation.

E. Cerebral venous thrombosis.

5.3 With regard to the treatment for intracranial hypotension, which one of the following statements is **TRUE**?

A. Conservative treatment for intracranial hypotension includes bed rest, hydration, and abdominal binders.

B. Surgical intervention is considered the mainstay of first-line interventional treatment.

C. Epidural blood patch is an alternative therapy if percutaneous placement of fibrin sealant proves ineffective.

D. The success rate of the first epidural blood patch is greater than 75%.

E. High-volume (20–100 mL) blood patches should be considered as the initial treatment in patients with cerebrospinal fluid (CSF) leaks.

Answers and Explanations

5.1   Correct: D. Intracranial hypotension.

This patient demonstrates classic signs of intracranial hypotension on magnetic resonance imaging (MRI) including bilateral subdural effusions, "sagging" of the brainstem, mild inferior displacement of the cerebellar tonsils, prominent pituitary gland, inferior displacement of the optic chiasm, diffuse dural enhancement, and engorged dural venous sinuses. Intracranial hypotension is a syndrome that is characterized by an orthostatic headache which is caused by reduced intracranial cerebrospinal fluid (CSF) pressure often due to a spontaneous spinal CSF leak. A good noninvasive study to identify spinal CSF leaks is computed tomography myelography. Most cases of spontaneous intracranial hypotension are self-limited, and the first line of treatment often involves conservative management with bed rest and hydration. However, depending on the severity and chronicity of symptoms, or for those with neurological symptoms or subdural hemorrhage, more aggressive management including epidural blood patch, percutaneous placement of fibrin sealant, and surgery may be necessary.

Other choices and discussion

A. The patient above has bilateral subdural effusions or hygromas, not bilateral subdural hematomas, in the setting of intracranial hypotension. However, subdural hematomas as well as hygromas are found in 15% of patients with intracranial hypotension. The presence of hemorrhage in patients with this disorder warrants more immediate consideration or application of an epidural blood patch.

B. Hypertrophic pachymeningitis is an uncommon disorder that causes a diffuse or localized thickening of the dura. It presents as diffuse dural thickening and enhancement on imaging. While this feature is present in this patient, other findings seen above such as bilateral subdural collections and brain sagging are not typical of this condition. Causes of hypertrophic pachymeningitis include trauma, infection, tumor, Wegener's granulomatosis, and IgG4-related autoimmune disease.

C. Chiari 1 malformation is characterized by elongated and peg-shaped cerebellar tonsils that extend below the foramen magnum with "crowding" of the posterior fossa and effacement of CSF spaces. Subdural collections, brain sagging, and diffuse dural enhancement are not observed with Chiari 1 malformation and can be used to differentiate this entity from intracranial hypotension. Mistaking Chiari 1 malformation for intracranial hypotension can be significant, as decompressive surgery for the former can exacerbate CSF leaks in patients with true intracranial hypotension.

E. Idiopathic intracranial hypertension is defined by increased intracranial pressure without an identifiable cause. Classic imaging features of this disorder include reduced pituitary height (with a partially empty or empty sella appearance), flattening of the posterior globe, intraocular protrusion of the optic nerve head, enlargement of the optic nerve sheath with prominence of the subarachnoid space around the nerves, tortuosity of the optic nerve, and cranial venous outflow obstruction including stenosis of the venous sinuses (most frequently involving the transverse sinuses). These features are not present in the above patient.

5.2   Correct: C. Disc-osteophyte.

Intracranial hypotension classically results from a spinal CSF leak. This may be related to a lumbar puncture, which introduces an iatrogenic tear in the dura and often causes transient CSF leaks. Spontaneous intracranial hypotension has been well-described in specific connective tissue disorders such as Ehler-Danlos syndrome type II and Marfan's syndrome, presumably due to defects of the extracellular matrix and its constituents such as fibrillin and microfils. Ruptured arachnoid diverticulum is a known cause of CSF leaks. Degenerative disc disease including disc herniations and osteophytes has been implicated as a cause of ventral spinal CSF leaks.

Other choices and discussion

A. There is a lack of evidence of an association between spontaneous intracranial hypotension and cranial CSF leaks. In fact, a spinal source of CSF leak should be sought in patients with orthostatic hypotension and a documented skull base CSF leak.

B, D. Intracranial hypotension has not been described in brain tumor or craniospin al irradiation unless a dural tear is present.

E. Cerebral venous thrombosis can be a complication, and is not a cause, of intracranial hypotension.

5.3   Correct: A. Conservative treatment for intracranial hypotension includes bed rest, hydration, and abdominal binders.

As most cases of spontaneous intracranial hypotension are self-limited, conservative management is thought to help relieve symptoms in most patients. The use of steroids, intravenous caffeine, or theophylline may also provide some added benefits. The injection of 10 to 20 mL of autologous blood into the spinal epidural space (epidural blood patch) is the mainstay of first-line interventional treatment. Symptomatic relief from the blood patch is thought to come as a result of the following three mechanisms: (1) blood volume replaces loss of CSF volume, (2) blood patch acts as a dural tamponade sealing the leak, and (3) blood restricts CSF flow within the epidural space and interferes with CSF absorption. It is not always necessary to inject the blood patch at the site of the leak, which is often unknown.

Other choices and discussion

D. The success rate with the first epidural blood patch used to treat patients with spontaneous intracranial hypotension is variable and ranges from 36 to 57% but it is not greater than 75%.

E. High-volume (20–100 mL) blood patches are generally considered in patients who have residual symptoms after treatment with first-time blood patch use (typically 10–20 mL).

C. Percutaneous placement of fibrin sealant is an alternative therapy if epidural blood patch proves ineffective and not the other way around. This procedure may be effective in one-third of patients in whom an epidural blood patch does not work. However, it requires being aware of the precise location of a CSF leak in order to maximize a successful outcome.

B. Surgical intervention should be considered in cases where the site of leak is clearly identified but response to conservative and minimally invasive interventions has been inadequate.

References

Graff-Radford SB, Schievink WI. High-pressure headaches, low-pressure syndromes, and CSF leaks: diagnosis and management. *Headache.* 2014;54:394–401.

Rohr AC, Riedel C, Fruehauf MC, et al. MR imaging findings in patients with secondary intracranial hypertension. AJNR Am *J Neuroradiol.* 2011;32:1021–1029.

Schievink WI1, Schwartz MS, Maya MM, et al. Lack of causal association between spontaneous intracranial hypotension and cranial cerebrospinal fluid leaks. *J Neurosurg.* 2012 Apr;116(4):749–754.

Su CS, Lan MY, Chang YY, et al. Clinical features, neuroimaging and treatment of spontaneous intracranial hypotension and magnetic resonance imaging evidence of blind epidural blood patch. *Eur Neurol.* 2009;61:301–307.

Case 6

Please refer to the following images to answer the next three questions:

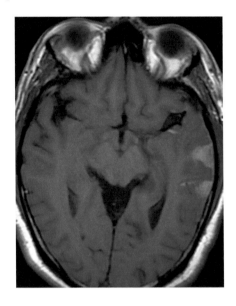 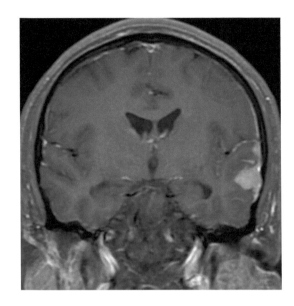

A 36-year-old male presents with new onset tonic–clonic seizures.

6.1 Which of the following **MOST** accurately characterizes the cause for the abnormal signal in the above lesion?

A. Fat.

B. Melanin.

C. Methemoglobin.

D. Manganese.

E. Contrast (gadolinium).

6.2 Which of the following statements is **TRUE** regarding primary central nervous system (CNS) melanoma?

A. Primary CNS melanoma is more common than secondary intracranial melanomas.

B. Primary leptomeningeal melanomatosis has a good prognosis.

C. Primary CNS melanoma is best diagnosed by histopathology.

D. Chemoradiation is the best treatment for primary CNs melanoma.

E. Primary melanocytic CNS tumors can present as a circumscribed mass or diffuse disease on imaging.

6.3 Which of the following is a rare congenital syndrome characterized by large and/or multiple melanocytic nevi of the skin and melanocytic lesions of the CNS?

A. Neurocutaneous melanosis.

B. Turcot syndrome.

C. Lynch syndrome.

D. Li-Fraumeni syndrome.

E. Gorlin syndrome.

Answers and Explanations

6.1 Correct: B. Melanin.

The paramagnetic properties of melanin result in characteristic hyperintensity on T1-weighted images and iso- or hypointensity on T2-weighted images. However, it is important to recognize that amelanotic lesions can show iso- to hypointensity on T1-weighted imaging and moderate hyperintensity on T2-weighted imaging. Furthermore, the presence of acute or chronic intratumoral bleeding may complicate evaluation of the lesion.

Other choices and discussion

A. Fat is not responsible for the signal abnormality in the above lesion for several reasons. On the first nonfat-suppressed image, there is intrinsic T1 hyperintense leptomeningeal signal and masses within the left temporal sulci. There is no evidence of chemical shift misregistration artifact, which is caused by differences in resonance frequencies of fat and water, to suggest the presence of fat within the lesions. This artifact manifests as a bright or dark outline at fat–water interfaces along the edge of an organ or lesion in the frequency-encoding direction. The lesion also remains T1 bright on the fat-saturated, postcontrast T1-weighted image (second image); therefore, as the signal is not nulled on this image, fat is not present within the lesion. Notably, fat suppression techniques help in minimizing or eliminating chemical shift artifacts.

C. There is no evidence of subacute hemorrhage (methemoglobin) in this patient. The imaging findings are consistent with a meningeal process that demonstrates T1 hyperintensity, most likely melanoma, given the mass-like appearance of the findings.

D. Manganese deposition due to chronic liver disease, total parenteral nutrition, or environmental exposures frequently present as T1 hyperintensity in the basal ganglia and not in the subarachnoid space.

E. The first image is prior to gadolinium administration, so contrast is not the cause for the hyperintense T1 signal abnormality in this patient.

6.2 Correct: E. Primary melanocytic CNS tumors can present as a circumscribed mass or diffuse disease on imaging.

Primary melanocytic tumors of the CNS, which are thought to arise from leptomeningeal melanocytes, include circumscribed masses such as melanocytoma (benign) and melanoma (malignant) as well as diffuse proliferations in the leptomeninges such as melanocytosis (benign) and melanomatosis (malignant). Circumscribed masses usually occur in adults, whereas diffuse diseases occur more often in children. The focal type has a generally better prognosis than the diffuse type because of the potential for complete excision of the former by surgery.

Other choices and discussion

A. Primary CNS melanoma is rare, accounting for about 1% of all cases of melanomas and less than 1% of all intracranial neoplasms. In contrast, secondary or metastatic melanomas are more common.

B. Primary leptomeningeal melanomatosis, a meningeal variant of primary intracranial malignant melanoma, is rare and has a poor prognosis. Depending on its location, it can present with symptoms of increased intracranial pressure or compression of anatomic structures due to obstruction of cerebrospinal fluid (CSF) flow at the basal cisterns and arachnoid granulations. It results from diffuse spread of malignant primary melanocytic cells along the leptomeninges with superficial invasion of the brain parenchyma.

C. The statement that primary CNS melanoma is best diagnosed by histopathology is false. As histopathological differentiation between primary and metastatic melanoma is difficult, primary CNS melanoma is usually diagnosed after the exclusion of a primary cutaneous, mucosal, or retinal malignant melanoma. Immunohistochemical, cytogenetic, and/or CSF studies all aid in the clinical diagnosis of this disease.

D. The best treatment for primary CNS melanoma is complete surgical excision if possible, and not chemoradiation, as melanoma is an aggressive and radioresistant tumor. In cases of complete excision, the prognosis is better with overall survival ranging from 1 to 28 years. Still, radiotherapy, chemotherapy, and/or immunotherapy techniques have been employed to prolong the lifespan of patients with melanoma and improve the control rate of lesions in the CNS.

6.3 Correct: A. Neurocutaneous melanosis.

Neurocutaneous melanosis is a congenital phakomatosis characterized by large and/or multiple melanocytic nevi of the skin and CNS melanocytic lesions, with the latter present in 40 to 60% of patients. These CNS lesions include leptomeningeal melanocytosis (benign) and leptomeningeal melanomatosis (malignant). The prognosis is very poor, especially when patients are symptomatic. Treatment including surgery, radiation, and chemotherapy is palliative with no significant impact on the clinical course.

Other choices and discussion

B. Turcot syndrome is an inherited disorder characterized by benign adenomatous polyps in the gastrointestinal tract and tumors of the CNS. The two most common types of brain tumors in this syndrome are glioblastoma and medulloblastoma.

C. Lynch syndrome, or hereditary nonpolyposis colorectal cancer, is an autosomal dominant condition characterized by an increased risk of developing multiple cancers including colon and other gastrointestinal types, endometrial, urinary tract, brain, and skin.

D. Li–Fraumeni syndrome is an autosomal dominant familial cancer syndrome characterized by an increased risk of developing sarcomas, breast cancer, leukemia, brain tumors, melanoma, and adrenal cortical tumors.

E. Gorlin syndrome, also known as basal cell nevus syndrome, is an autosomal dominant tumor syndrome characterized by multiple basal cell carcinomas, odontogenic keratocysts, dural calcifications, ovarian and cardiac fibromas, and medulloblastomas.

References

Ko CC, Tai MH, Li CF, et al. Differentiation between Glioblastoma Multiforme and Primary Cerebral Lymphoma: Additional Benefits of Quantitative Diffusion-Weighted MR Imaging. *PLoS ONE*. 2016;11(9):e0162565.

Mansour A, Qandeel M, Abdel-Razeq H, et al. MR imaging features of intracranial primary CNS lymphoma in immune competent patients. *Cancer Imaging*. 2014;14:22.

Osborn AG, Salzman KL, Jhaveri MD. *Diagnostic Imaging: Brain*. 3rd ed. Elsevier; 2016:566–569.

Toh CH, Castillo M, Wong AM, et al. Primary cerebral lymphoma and glioblastoma multiforme: differences in diffusion characteristics evaluated with diffusion tensor imaging. *AJNR Am J Neuroradiol*. 2008;29(3):471–475.

Case 7

Please refer to the following images to answer the next three questions:

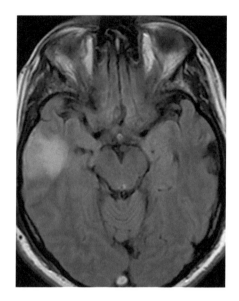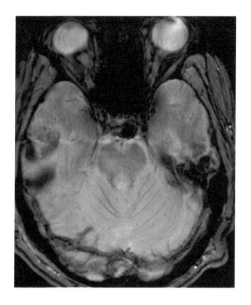

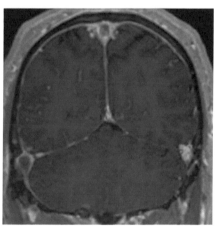

A 40-year-old male presents with headache.

7.1 What is the **MOST** likely diagnosis?

A. Astrocytoma.
B. Focal cortical dysplasia.
C. Invasive fungal infection.
D. Right middle cerebral artery infarction.
E. Hemorrhagic venous infarction.

7.2 Which of the following is a sign of venous sinus thrombosis on contrast-enhanced computed tomography (CT)?

A. Triangle sign.
B. Empty delta sign.

C. Cord sign.
D. Medusa head sign.
E. Insular ribbon sign.

7.3 What is the imaging hallmark of thrombosis of the internal cerebral veins, vein of Galen, or straight sinus?

A. Dural arteriovenous fistula.
B. Thalamic enhancement.
C. Intraventricular hemorrhage.
D. Thalamic hemorrhage.
E. Thalamic edema.

Answers and Explanations

7.1 Correct: E. Hemorrhagic venous infarction.

As many as 57% of patients with cerebral venous thrombosis have parenchymal abnormalities, including focal vasogenic and/or cytotoxic edema and hemorrhage, which often but not always occur in areas of the brain that are drained directly by the occluded venous sinus. A filling defect in or occlusion of the dural venous sinuses on computed tomography or magnetic resonance venography, or 3D volumetric, postcontrast T1-weighted images, is the key to the diagnosis. In contrast to arterial infarcts, parenchymal abnormalities, due to venous thrombosis, are typically reversible, although areas of cytotoxic edema (manifested by the presence of restricted diffusion) may be permanent. The enhancement of the cortex, tentorium, and leptomeninges may also be present. While the mechanism of hemorrhage in venous thrombosis is multifactorial, it is likely related to continued arterial perfusion in areas of dead tissue as well as elevation of venous pressures beyond the capacity of the venous wall. In the case presented above, a filling defect is seen within the right transverse sinus on the postcontrast coronal image (second image); consequently, there is edema (first image) in the right temporal lobe, which is consistent with venous infarction.

Other choices and discussion

A–D. The other answer choices like astrocytoma, focal cortical dysplasia, invasive fungal infection, and right middle cerebral artery infarction would not produce this constellation of imaging findings and are therefore incorrect. While invasive fungal infections such as cerebral aspergillosis or mucormycosis can produce hemorrhagic infarct-like lesions, no other imaging or clinical findings to support infection are present. Also, the patient is neither immunocompromised nor diabetic, both of which are risk factors contributing to disseminated fungal infection.

7.2 Correct: B. Empty delta sign.

The empty delta sign indicates cerebral venous sinus occlusive disease, most often involving the superior sagittal sinus, and refers to a central filling defect (thrombus) within a dural sinus and with a surrounding triangular area of contrast-enhancement (dural collateral venous channels). It is only described with contrast-enhanced CT or magnetic resonance imaging and not with noncontrast studies.

Other choices and discussion

A. The triangle sign is a sign of dural sinus thrombosis on noncontrast CT. It represents clotted blood within the superior sagittal sinus, which appears hyperdense.
C. The cord sign is a sign of venous thrombosis on noncontrast CT. It represents a cord-like hyperdensity within a cortical vein or dural sinus.
D. Medusa head sign refers to the multiple venous tributaries of a developmental venous anomaly which are arranged in a radial fashion and ultimately drain into a larger draining vein.
E. The insular ribbon sign refers to the loss of the normal gray–white differentiation of the insula and is one of the earliest imaging signs of middle cerebral artery territory infarction.

7.3 Correct: E. Thalamic edema.

Thalamic edema is identified in over 75% of patients with thrombosis of the internal cerebral veins, vein of Galen, and/or straight sinus on computed tomography and magnetic resonance imaging. The edema is typically bilateral, although unilateral edema may occur. Over half of the patients afflicted with this specific condition have no neurologic sequelae.

Other choices and discussion

A. While cerebral venous occlusive disease may be an underlying etiologic factor for the development of dural arteriovenous fistulas, this is not a classic imaging finding for internal cerebral vein, vein of Galen, or straight sinus thrombosis.
B–D. Thalamic enhancement and intraventricular hemorrhage are not the hallmark features of this condition. Hemorrhage is present in approximately 20% of patients with thrombosis of the internal cerebral veins, vein of Galen, and/or straight sinus, and is typically located in the thalami.

References

Chavhan GB, Shroff MM. Twenty classic signs in neuroradiology: A pictorial essay. *Indian J Radiol Imaging.* 2009;19:135–145.

Leach JL, Fortuna RB, Jones BV, et al. Imaging of cerebral venous thrombosis: current techniques, spectrum of findings, and diagnostic pitfalls. *Radiographics.* 2006;26 (Suppl 1):S19–S41.

Rodallec MH, Krainik A, Feydy A, et al. Cerebral venous thrombosis and multidetector CT angiography: tips and tricks. *Radiographics.* 2006;26(Suppl 1):S5–S18.

Case 8

Please refer to the following images to answer the next three questions:

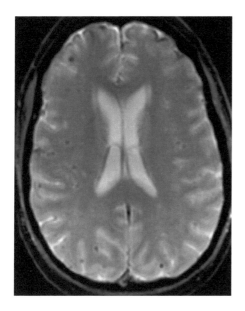

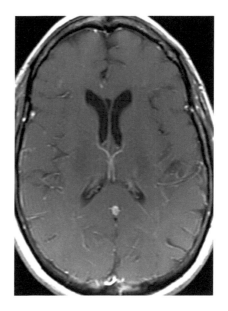

A 78-year-old male presents with progressive cognitive decline.

8.1 Which is the **MOST** likely diagnosis?

A. Metastatic d isease.

B. Diffuse axonal injury (DAI).

C. Neurocysticercosis.

D. Multiple cerebral cavernous malformations (CCM).

E. Cerebral amyloid angiopathy (CAA).

8.2 What is the **MOST** common presentation of symptomatic cerebral amyloid angiopathy (CAA)?

A. Seizure.

B. Rapidly progressive dementia.

C. Intracerebral hemorrhage.

D. Fatigue.

E. Parkinsonism.

8.3 What is the **MOST** important risk factor contributing to the development of CAA?

A. Hypertension.

B. Increasing age.

C. Type II diabetes.

D. Smoking.

E. Male gender.

Answers and Explanations

8.1 Correct: E. Cerebral amyloid angiopathy (CAA).

The patient in the above case has multiple gradient echo (GRE) hypointense foci throughout the brain parenchyma, predominantly located in the peripheral brain, as well as leptomeningeal hemosiderin staining in the frontal lobes without associated enhancement. Given the age of this patient (>60 years old) and lack of cancer history or trauma, the most likely diagnosis is cerebral amyloid angiopathy. CAA is the consequence of beta–amyloid deposition in the walls of cortical and leptomeningeal blood vessels. Most patients have multifocal and confluent areas of T2 hyperintense signal in the supratentorial white matter, which are nonspecific, but some will also have primarily supratentorial and peripheral cerebral microhemorrhages and cortical superficial siderosis, which aid in the diagnosis. Up to 50% of individuals over 80 years of age display some pathologic evidence of CAA as part of the normal aging process, but other patients with CAA can have symptoms.

Other choices and discussion

A. Metastases can exhibit hypointense signal on blood-sensitive sequences such as GRE or susceptibility-weighted imaging due to hemorrhage, tumoral calcification, or calcification related to treatment. Radiation therapy can also result in hypointensites related to radiation-induced capillary telangiectasias and cavernous malformations. Metastases, however, often enhance following contrast administration, which is absent in this case.

B. Diffuse axonal injury results in multifocal shear injuries situated in the subcortical white matter, corpus callosum, and dorsal brainstem. Shear injuries may be hemorrhagic and are best depicted on blood-sensitive sequences or may be nonhemorrhagic and are best depicted on diffusion-weighted imaging sequence. Concomitant post-traumatic subarachnoid hemorrhage could account for leptomeningeal T2* hypointensity. This is not the best answer choice, however, as there is no history of trauma.

C. Multiple parenchymal calcifications seen in the calcified nodular stage of neurocysticercosis can produce numerous hypointense signal foci in the brain on T2* sequences. However, one would not expect linear hypointense signal in the leptomeninges. The classic cavernous malformation is a lobulated ("popcorn" or "mulberry") lesion containing locules of variable T2 and T1 signal due to blood products of varying ages, and a hemosiderin rim of marked T2* hypointensity.

D. In familial cases of cavernous malformations, the lesions may be tiny, appearing only as multiple small foci of hypointensity on T2*. While the imaging findings could be compatible with cerebral cavernous malformations, the hypointense signal in the leptomeninges and the clinical history suggest a different diagnosis.

8.2 Correct: C. Intracerebral hemorrhage.

CAA accounts for 5 to 20% of spontaneous intracerebral hemorrhages in the elderly and is the most dramatic clinical presentation of this condition.

Other choices and discussion

A. Seizure is not the most common presentation, although it may occur in the context of acute intracerebral hemorrhage. CAA is associated with dementia and cognitive impairment.

B. *Rapidly progressive* dementia is relatively rare. This latter clinical phenotype is associated with CAA-related inflammation, the imaging findings of which are large confluent areas of asymmetric T2 hyperintense signal in the cerebral white matter, with little if any mass effect.

D, E. The presence of the typical microhemorrhages seen in CAA can aid in the diagnosis, but they are not always present. CAA is not associated with parkinsonism or fatigue.

8.3 Correct: B. Increasing age.

Advancing age is the strongest risk factor contributing to the development of CAA.

Other choices and discussion

A. Hypertension need not be present in patients with CAA; it can be seen in normotensive patients. While there exists some evidence to suggest that controlling hypertension may decrease the risk of intracerebral hemorrhage (ICH) in patients with CAA, hypertension does not appear to be a risk factor contributing to the development of CAA.

C. CAA has been associated with type II diabetes but this is not the most important risk factor.

D. Smoking is not a risk factor contributing to the development of CAA.

E. There does not appear to be a strong gender predilection for CAA.

References

Biffi A, Greenberg SM. Cerebral amyloid angiopathy: a systematic review. *J Clin Neurol.* 2011;7:1–9.

Linn J, Herms J, Dichgans M, et al. Subarachnoid hemosiderosis and superficial cortical hemosiderosis in cerebral amyloid angiopathy. AJNR *Am J Neuroradiol.* 2008;29:184–186.

Osborn AG. Osborn's brain: imaging, pathology, and anatomy. Wolters Kluwer/Lippincott Williams & Wilkins, 2012.

Case 9

Please refer to the following images to answer the next three questions:

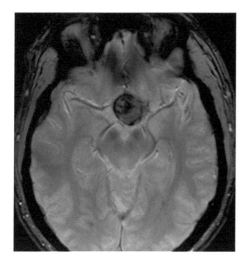
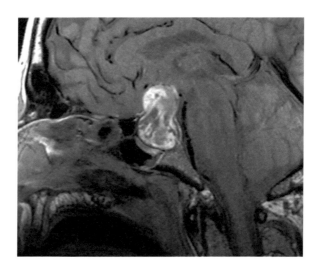

A 50-year-old male presents with headache and decreased visual acuity.

9.1 What is the **MOST** likely diagnosis?

A. Rathke cleft cyst.

B. Meningioma.

C. Craniopharyngioma.

D. Hemorrhagic pituitary adenoma.

E. Aneurysm.

9.2 What clinical syndrome does the patient have?

A. Kallman syndrome.

B. Sheehan syndrome.

C. Pituitary apoplexy.

D. Parinaud syndrome.

E. Wallenberg syndrome.

9.3 Which of the following is the **MOST** common symptom of pituitary apoplexy?

A. Headache.

B. Diplopia.

C. Altered mental status.

D. Adrenal insufficiency.

E. Cortical blindness.

Answers and Explanations

9.1 Correct: D. Hemorrhagic pituitary adenoma.

The images demonstrate a sellar lesion with suprasellar extension and remodeling of the sella turcica. A normal pituitary gland cannot be identified. The lesion is hemorrhagic, as demonstrated by the low signal on the gradient echo image and heterogeneously hyperintense signal on the noncontrast T1-weighted image. Most cases of pituitary hemorrhage are due to an underlying pituitary macroadenoma; although less frequently, hemorrhage can be seen in other lesions and histologically normal glands. In this case, a pituitary adenoma was found at surgery.

Other choices and discussion

A. Rathke cleft cysts are nonenhancing lesions with variable but usually homogeneous signal intensity on T1- and T2-weighted imaging. They are classically midline in location and closely associated with the posterior gland. A characteristic T2 hypointense nodule within the cyst can be observed.
B. Meningiomas are enhancing masses that are isointense to gray matter on T1- and T2-weighted images. In the setting of a meningioma, the pituitary gland should be identifiable as a separate structure from the mass.
C. Craniopharyngiomas are generally suprasellar tumors that have mixed cystic and solid components and calcification. Identification of the pituitary gland as a separate structure from the mass is also expected with a craniopharyngioma. Craniopharyngiomas can occur in both pediatric and middle-aged adults. The adamantinomatous subtype seen in children is classically cystic-solid on imaging and may calcify, and the papillary subtype that can be seen in adults is more solid and does not calcify.
E. Although aneurysm is in the differential for a suprasellar mass, the expansion of the sella (due to a slowly growing pituitary mass), no separately identified pituitary gland (suggesting that the mass is pituitary in origin), and no contiguity of the sellar/suprasellar mass with a vessel in this case argues against aneurysm.

9.2 Correct: C. Pituitary apoplexy.

Pituitary apoplexy is the acute clinical syndrome of headache, visual deficits, and endocrinologic deficiencies associated with hemorrhage into, or infarction of, the pituitary gland. An underlying macroadenoma is often the culprit. While hemorrhage is commonly found in macroadenomas, clinical pituitary apoplexy occurs in only a small proportion of patients with pituitary adenomas (1–9%).

Other choices and discussion

A. Kallman syndrome is a genetic syndrome manifested by idiopathic hypogonadotrophic gonadism and anosmia. Imaging demonstrates hypoplasia or aplasia of the olfactory bulbs and structural changes of the basal forebrain.
B. Sheehan syndrome is a variant of pituitary apoplexy. Specifically, it refers to infarction of the adenohypophysis due to hypovolemic shock from excessive blood loss during or following childbirth.
D. Parinaud syndrome is vertical gaze palsy associated with a pineal tumor.
E. Wallenberg syndrome is a consequence of a lateral medullary infarct and is manifested by loss of contralateral body pain and temperature sensation, loss of ipsilateral facial pain and temperature sensation, and ipsilateral Horner's syndrome.

9.3 Correct: A. Headache.

Headache is the most common symptom of pituitary apoplexy and occurs in nearly 100% of patients with this condition.

Other choices and discussion

B. Diplopia is not the most common symptom of pituitary apoplexy but occurs frequently (in approximately 70% of patients). Sudden enlargement of tissue in the sella turcica from hemorrhage can result in ocular paresis and diplopia due to mass effect upon cranial nerves in the cavernous sinus.
C. Altered mental status can occur in up to 30% patients with pituitary apoplexy. Adrenocorticotropic hormone (ACTH) is secreted by the pituitary gland and stimulates cortisol secretion from the adrenal gland.
D. Pituitary apoplexy can result in acute adrenal insufficiency with life-threatening hypotension, but this is not the most common manifestation.
E. Cortical blindness is a result of bilateral occipital lobe lesions and does not result from pituitary apoplexy.

References

Bonneville JF, Bonneville F, Cattin F. Magnetic resonance imaging of pituitary adenomas. **Eur Radiol**. 2005;15:543–548.

Byun WM, Kim OL, Kim D. MR imaging findings of Rathke's cleft cysts. *AJNR Am J Neuroradiol*. 2000;21:485–488.

Osborn AG. Osborn's Brain: Imaging, Pathology, and Anatomy. Wolters Kluwer/Lippincott Williams & Wilkins, 2012.

Wenya LB, Dunn IF, Laws ER. Pituitary Apoplexy. *Endocrine*. 2015;48:69–75.

Case 10

Please refer to the following images to answer the next three questions:

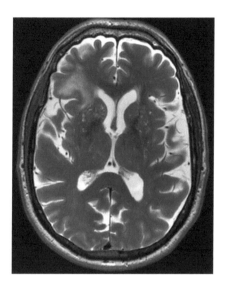 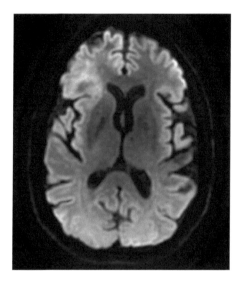

A 60-year-old male with history of recurrent lymphoma treated with rituximab presents with slurred speech.

10.1 What is the **MOST** likely diagnosis?

A. Central nervous system (CNS) cryptococcosis.

B. Cytomegalovirus (CMV) ventriculoencephalitis.

C. Herpes simplex virus (HSV) encephalitis.

D. Progressive multifocal leukoencephalopathy (PML).

E. Toxoplasmosis.

10.2 Which of the following microorganism is responsible for PML?

A. JC polyomavirus.

B. Hantavirus.

C. Epstein–Barr virus.

D. Prions.

E. Blastomyces dermatitidis.

10.3 In what situation might you see robust contrast enhancement associated with progressive multifocal leukoencephalopathy (PML) lesions?

A. Organ transplant recipient with new diagnosis of PML.

B. Patient with acute myeloid leukemia and new diagnosis of PML.

C. Patient with HIV and new diagnosis of PML.

D. Patient with dermatomyositis and new diagnosis of PML.

E. Patient with multiple sclerosis on natalizumab and diagnosis of PML.

Answers and Explanations

10.1 Correct: D. Progressive multifocal leukoencephalopathy (PML).

Imaging findings of PML include white matter lesions involving the subcortical U-fibers that exhibit restricted diffusion along the periphery and have minimal mass effect. This appearance in an immunocompromised patient should highly raise the suspicion of PML, which is caused by reactivation of the human polyomavirus JC in the setting of immunosupression. The parietal lobe is most frequently involved, followed by the frontal, temporal, and occipital lobes. Posterior fossa involvement is less frequent; if present, the cerebellar hemispheric white matter is typically involved.

Other choices and discussion

A. CNS cryptococcosis manifests as meningitis with leptomeningeal enhancement, gelatinous pseudocysts with cystic expansion of the perivascular spaces in the brain (especially in the basal ganglia), and cryptococcomas with focal-enhancing lesions in the brain. In immunocompromised patients, reactivation of CMV can result in disseminated infection. In the CNS, this can manifest as ventriculoencephalitis, meningoencephalitis, retinitis, myelitis, and polyradiculitis.
B. MRI in CMV ventriculoencephalitis can demonstrate subependymal restricted diffusion, fluid-attenuated inversion recovery (FLAIR) hyperintensity, and enhancement.
C. HSV encephalitis involves the temporal lobes, inferior frontal lobes, insula, and cingulate gyri. Involvement is typically asymmetric when bilateral. MRI demonstrates edema in the affected regions and may show areas of restricted diffusion and hemorrhage. Enhancement is variable. Absence of mesial temporal lobe involvement in the above case argues against HSV encephalitis.
E. CNS toxoplasmosis typically presents as multiple solidly enhancing lesions, ring-enhancing lesions, or ring-enhancing lesions with an associated eccentric solid nodule ("eccentric target sign"). The lesions have a predilection for the deep gray matter structures and the gray–white junction.

10.2 Correct: A. JC polyomavirus.

The JC virus is a human polyomavirus that causes progressive multifocal leukoencephalopathy (PML) in immunocompromised patients, such as patients with a hematological malignancy or HIV and solid organ transplant recipients. Specific drugs such as rituximab and natalizumab have resulted in PML in patients treated with these agents and are, therefore, contraindicated in those who are infected.

Other choices and discussion

B. Hantavirus is a member of the bunyavirus family that causes Hantavirus hemorrhagic fever with renal syndrome and Hantavirus pulmonary syndrome or Hantavirus cardiopulmonary syndrome.

C. Epstein-Barr virus, also known as human herpesvirus 4, is the underlying pathogen of infectious mononucleosis, and can also cause diseases that affect the central nervous system such as encephalitis, meningitis, acute disseminated encephalomyelitis, seizures, polyradiculomyelitis, cranial nerve palsies, and transverse myelitis.
D. A prion is a transmissible protein that causes abnormal folding of normal cellular proteins in the brain. Prions are responsible for progressive neurodegenerative disorders such as Creutzfeldt-Jakob disease.
E. *Blastomyces dermatitidis* is a dimorphic fungus that causes blastomycosis, which is an infection that can involve multiple organs in the body such as the lungs, skin, bone, genitourinary system, and the central nervous system.

10.3 Correct: E. Patient with multiple sclerosis on natalizumab and diagnosis of PML.

Classic PML lesions generally do not enhance, except in the setting of immune reconstitution inflammatory syndrome (IRIS-PML). In patients with HIV and PML, this occurs within weeks, months, and, rarely, years after highly active antiretroviral therapy (HAART) is initiated. IRIS-PML can also occur in multiple sclerosis patients on natalizumab therapy who can develop PML within days to weeks after plasma exchange is initiated. Patients present with clinical deterioration, and on imaging, develop increased size of, and edema and enhancement associated with, their lesions. The other choices reflect new diagnoses of PML in the absence of immune reconstitution and are incorrect.

Other choices and discussion

A–D. Organ transplant recipients, patients with hematologic malignances such as acute myeloid leukemia, patients with HIV, and patients with autoimmune disease such as dermatomyositis, however, are populations at risk of contracting PML.

References

Bergui M, Bradac GB, Oguz KK, et al. Progressive multifocal lekoencephalopathy: diffusion-weighted imaging and pathological correlations. *Neuroradiology*. 2004;46:22–25.

Clifford DB, DeLuca A, Simpson DM, et al. Natalizumab-associated progressive multifocal leukoencephalopathy in patients with multiple sclerosis: lessons from 28 cases. *Lancet Neurol*. 2010;9:438–446.

Post MJD, Thurnher MM, Clifford DB, et al. CNS-immune reconstitution inflammatory syndrome in the setting of HIV infection, part 1: Overview and discussion of progressive multifocal leukoencephalopathy-immune reconstitution inflammatory syndrome and cryptococcal-immune reconstitution inflammatory syndrome. *AJNR Am J Neuroradiol*. 2013; 34:1297–1307.

Rath TJ, Hughes M, Arabi M, et al. Imaging of cerebritis, encephalitis, and brain abscess. *Neuroimag Clin N Am*. 2012; 22:585–607.

Case 11

Please refer to the following images to answer the next three questions:

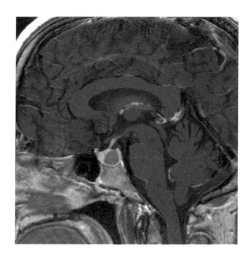
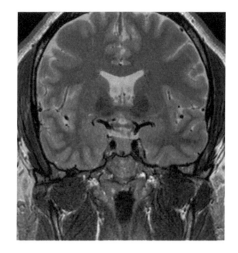

A 33-year-old male presents with decreased libido, depression, and headache.

11.1 What is the **MOST** likely diagnosis?

A. Craniopharyngioma.

B. Pituitary adenoma.

C. Arachnoid cyst.

D. Rathke cleft cyst.

E. Lymphocytic hypophysitis.

11.2 What is the tissue of origin of this lesion?

A. Notochordal rests.

B. Ventral diencephalon.

C. Craniopharyngeal canal.

D. Meninx primitiva.

E. Oral ectoderm.

11.3 What is the most common sign or symptom associated with a RCC?

A. Visual field defect.

B. Headache.

C. Pituitary dysfunction.

D. Pituitary apoplexy.

E. Meningismus.

Answers and Explanations

11.1 Correct: D. Rathke cleft cyst.

Magnetic resonance images show a nonenhancing T2 hyperintense cystic lesion located between the anterior and posterior lobes of the pituitary gland, containing an intracystic T2 hypointense nodule. The imaging findings are consistent with a Rathke cleft cyst (RCC). RCCs arise from the vestigial intermediate lobe of the pituitary gland and as a result usually occupy a strictly midline location, although off-midline and suprasellar locations can (uncommonly) occur. The imaging appearance is influenced by the composition of the cyst contents, although the lesion is usually hyperattenuating on CT; on MRI, the lesion is T1 hypo to hyperintense and usually T2 hyperintense. The characteristic nonenhancing T1 hyperintense and T2 hypointense intracystic nodule is seen in up to 75% of RCCs. RCCs lack enhancement and usually lack calcification, and the presence of either feature should lead one to consider alterative diagnoses.

Other choices and discussion

A. Craniopharyngiomas are cystic suprasellar neoplasms that can extend into the sella. The presence of an enhancing soft-tissue component and calcification aid in distinguishing these lesions from RCCs.

B. Pituitary adenomas can be cystic and may be difficult to distinguish from RCCs when there is no identifiable, enhancing soft-tissue component on imaging. They, however, lack the nonenhancing intracystic nodule characteristic of RCC.

C. Arachnoid cysts in this region present as cystic sellar lesions with suprasellar extension, which follow cerebrospinal fluid (CSF)-signal intensity and displace and compress normal pituitary gland.

E. Lymphocytic hypophysitis is characterized by infiltration of the pituitary stalk and/or pituitary gland by inflammatory cells and most frequently affects peripartum women. Imaging features include thickening of the pituitary stalk, loss of the normal posterior pituitary bright spot, and enlargement of the pituitary gland.

11.2 Correct: E. Oral ectoderm.

Rathke cleft cysts (RCCs) arise from remnants of Rathke's pouch, which is derived embryologically from the thickening of cells in the oral ectoderm and is referred to as the hypophyseal placode.

Other choices and discussion

A. Notochordal rests are the presumed tissue of origin of chordomas.

C. The craniopharyngeal canal is a defect in the sphenoid bone, extending between the floor of the sella turcica to the nasopharynx, and is thought to result from incomplete closure of Rathke's pouch.

B. The downward extension of the ventral diencephalon forms the posterior lobe of the pituitary gland.

D. The meninx primitiva is the mesenchymal embryologic structure that gives rise to the meninges.

11.3 Correct: B. Headache.

Headache is the most common symptom observed in patients with RCC and may be the only symptom in 40% of cases.

Other choices and discussion

A, C. Visual field disturbance and pituitary dysfunction are also associated with RCC but are less common than headache.

D, E. Acute presentations such as apoplexy which are secondary to intracystic hemorrhage with rapid lesion, enlargement, and meningismus, due to cyst rupture and spillage of cyst fluid into the subarachnoid space are rare.

References

Bergui M, Bradac GB, Oguz KK, et al. Progressive multifocal lekoencephalopathy: diffusion-weighted imaging and pathological correlations. *Neuroradiology.* 2004;46:22–25.

Clifford DB, DeLuca A, Simpson DM, et al. Natalizumab-associated progressive multifocal leukoencephalopathy in patients with multiple sclerosis: lessons from 28 cases. *Lancet Neurol.* 2010;9:438–446.

Post MJD, Thurnher MM, Clifford DB, et al. CNS-immune reconstitution inflammatory syndrome in the setting of HIV infection, part 1: Overview and discussion of progressive multifocal leukoencephalopathy-immune reconstitution inflammatory syndrome and cryptococcal-immune reconstitution inflammatory syndrome. *AJNR Am J Neuroradiol.* 2013; 34:1297–1307

Rath TJ, Hughes M, Arabi M, et al. Imaging of cerebritis, encephalitis, and brain abscess. *Neuroimag Clin N Am.* 2012; 22:585–607.

Case 12

Please refer to the following images to answer the next three questions:

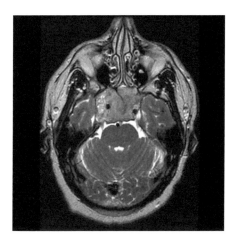

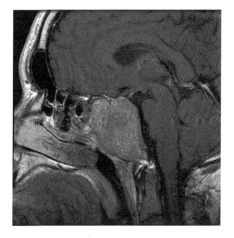

A 52-year-old male with a history of erectile dysfunction and low testosterone was found to have a prolactin level of 28,000 ng/mL.

12.1 What is the **MOST** likely diagnosis based on the imaging findings and the clinical information?

A. Chordoma.

B. Metastasis.

C. Pituitary adenoma.

D. Meningioma.

E. Plasmacytoma.

12.2 What preoperative MRI feature is **MOST** predictive of incomplete excision of the parasellar component of a pituitary adenoma?

A. Asymmetry of the cavernous sinuses.

B. Displacement of the cavernous internal carotid artery (ICA).

C. Less than 50% encasement of the cavernous ICA.

D. Involvement of the inferolateral or lateral venous compartments of the cavernous sinus.

E. Involvement of the superior venous compartment of the cavernous sinus.

12.3 Which of the following is the **MOST** common type of pituitary adenoma?

A. Nonfunctioning adenoma.

B. Prolactinoma.

C. Somatotroph adenoma.

D. Corticotroph adenoma.

E. Thyrotroph adenoma.

Answers and Explanations

12.1 Correct: C. Pituitary adenoma.

Axial T2-weighted and sagittal postcontrast T1-weighted images show a soft tissue mass centered in the sphenoid bone, extending laterally into the cavernous sinuses where it encases the right cavernous internal carotid artery flow void. There is involvement of the clivus posteriorly and extension into the nasopharynx anteriorly. Importantly, there is contiguous soft tissue in the sella and no normal pituitary gland is observed. This key feature distinguishes invasive pituitary adenomas from other invasive central skull base lesions.

Other choices and discussion

A. Chordomas are lytic tumors that arise from notochordal rests in the skull base or spine. They are typically hyperintense on T2-weighted images, exhibit restricted diffusion, and have variable degrees and patterns of contrast enhancement.

B. Metastases should be suspected if multiple lesions are present or if there is a history of malignancy.

D. Central skull base meningiomas are centered upon dural surfaces (look for a dural tail!) and would not replace the pituitary gland.

E. Plasmacytomas exhibit homogeneous low-to-intermediate T2 signal intensity and may be seen as a solitary lesion or can occur in the setting of multiple myelomatous lesions.

12.2 Correct: D. Involvement of the inferolateral or lateral venous compartments of the cavernous sinus.

Parasellar involvement by pituitary adenomas occurs in 6 to 10% of cases and increases the likelihood of incomplete surgical resection and requirement for additional therapy. Involvement of the (1) inferolateral or (2) lateral venous compartments of the cavernous sinus (in relation to the cavernous internal carotid artery) and (3) encasement of the cavernous internal carotid artery by *greater than* 50% are indicators that the parasellar component of the adenoma is unlikely to be resected.

Other choices and discussion

C. Less than 50% encasement of the cavernous internal carotid artery, is false.

E, B, and **A.** Involvement of the superior venous compartment of the cavernous sinus, displacement of the cavernous ICA, and asymmetry of the cavernous sinuses are less strongly predictive features of incomplete parasellar tumor resection.

12.3 Correct: B. Prolactinoma.

Prolactinomas comprise 30 to 45% of pituitary adenomas and are the most common type.

Other choices and discussion

A, C–E. Nonfunctioning adenomas comprise 25 to 35%, somatotroph adenomas 15%, corticotroph adenomas 10%, and thyrotroph adenomas 1%.

References

Connor SEJ, Wilson F, Hogarth K. Magnetic Resonance Imaging Criteria to Predict Complete Excision of Parasellar Pituitary Macroadenoma on Postoperative Imaging. *J Neurol Surg B Skull Base.* 2014;75(1):41–46.

Louis RG, Dallapiazza R, Jane Jr . JA. Chapter 10: Sellar Tumors: Pituitary Adenomas and Craniopharyngiomas. In: Packer RJ, Schiff D, eds. *Neuro-oncology, First Edition.* Chichester, West Sussex: Wiley-Blackwell; 2012.

Case 13

Please refer to the following images to answer the next three questions:

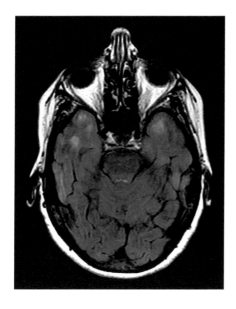

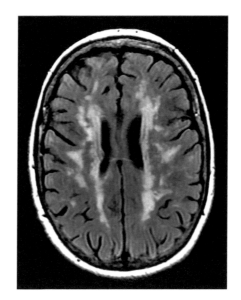

A 58-year-old male with a strong family history of dementia presents with mild cognitive impairment.

13.1 What is the **MOST** likely diagnosis?

A. MELAS (mitochondrial encephalomyopathy, lactic acidosis, and stroke-like episodes).

B. Creutzfeldt-Jakob disease.

C. CADASIL (cerebral autosomal dominant arteriopathy with subcortical infarcts and leukoencephalopathy).

D. Alzheimer's disease (AD).

E. Multiple sclerosis (MS).

13.2 What further testing will confirm the diagnosis of CADASIL (cerebral autosomal dominant arteriopathy with subcortical infarcts and leukoencephalopathy)?

A. Genetic testing for NOTCH3 mutation.

B. RT-QuIC anaylsis of cerebrospinal fluid (CSF).

C. CSF analysis for oligoclonal bands.

D. Positron emission tomography (PET) scan for amyloid plaque detection.

E. Genetic testing for mitochondrial mutation.

13.3 Which imaging pattern is most suggestive of CADASIL (cerebral autosomal dominant arteriopathy with subcortical infarcts and leukoencephalopathy)?

A. Cortical ribboning on diffusion-weighted imaging (DWI).

B. Temporo-parietal predominant atrophy.

C. Multiple nonterritorial strokes of different ages.

D. Diffuse white matter T2 signal abnormality with anterior temporal subcortical involvement.

E. Multiple white matter T2 signal abnormalities, many ovoid and perpendicularly oriented to the corpus callosum.

Answers and Explanations

13.1 Correct: C. CADASIL (cerebral autosomal dominant arteriopathy with subcortical infarcts and leukoencephalopathy).

Extensive white matter signal abnormality with prominent anterior temporal involvement in a patient with family history of dementia is most suggestive of CADASIL. CADASIL is a genetic, nonatherosclerotic small vessel vasculopathy which usually presents in the third or fourth decade of life, and is the most common genetic cause of subcortical vascular dementia. It is caused by a mutation in the NOTCH3 gene on chromosome 19. Involvement of the anterior temporal subcortical white matter is an early and prominent finding, with more common involvement of the periventricular white matter, external capsule, and corpus callosum as the disease progresses.

Other choices and discussion

A. MELAS presents in childhood or early adulthood with infarct-like cortical lesions which cross vascular territories. Diagnosis is made by genetic testing for mitochondrial mutations.

B. Creutzfeldt-Jakob disease is characterized by progressive restricted diffusion in the cerebral cortex and deep gray nuclei ("cortical ribboning"). Diagnosis can be confirmed by real-time quaking-induced conversion (RT-QuIC) of cerebrospinal fluid (CSF) to detect the presence of pathologic prion protein.

D. AD may show temporoparietal predominant volume loss, but no specific MRI findings may be present and anterior temporal white signal abnormality is not typical. Nuclear medicine scans are helpful, with amyloid plaque positron emission tomography (PET) most useful for excluding AD and perfusion single-photon emission computed tomography (SPECT) showing temporoparietal hypoperfusion.

E. Anterior temporal white matter lesions may be seen in MS. However, MS is a less likely differential consideration for this case, as MS is more common in middle-aged patients. MS white matter lesions are perpendicularly oriented to the corpus callosum, and active lesions demonstrate peripheral or incomplete rim enhancement. In addition, detection of oligoclonal bands in the CSF may aid in the diagnosis of MS.

13.2 Correct: A. Genetic testing for NOTCH3 mutation.

Genetic testing for NOTCH3 mutation confirms a diagnosis of CADASIL.

Other choices and discussion

B–E. These choices are incorrect, see discussion in the previous question.

13.3 Correct: D. Diffuse white matter T2 signal abnormality with anterior temporal subcortical involvement.

T2 hyperintense signal abnormality in the anterior temporal subcortical white matter is an early and prominent finding of CADASIL, with involvement of the periventricular white matter, external capsule, and corpus callosum found with disease progression.

Other choices and discussion

A. Cortical ribboning on DWI is a typical finding of Creutzfeldt-Jakob disease.

B. Temporoparietal predominant atrophy may be present in advanced Alzheimer's disease (AD), although no specific findings of AD are commonly present on structural MRI.

C. Multiple nonterritorial strokes of different ages is a finding of MELAS (mitochondrial encephalomyopathy, lactic acidosis, and stroke-like episodes).

E. Ovoid white matter lesions oriented perpendicularly to the corpus callosum described as "Dawson's fingers," are classic imaging appearance of multiple sclerosis lesions.

References

Sarbu N, Shih RY, Jones RV, et al. White Matter Diseases with Radiologic-Pathologic Correlation. *Radiographics*. 2016;36(5):1426–1447.

Singhal S, Rich P, Markus HS. The spatial distribution of MR imaging abnormalities in cerebral autosomal dominant arteriopathy with subcortical infarcts and leukoencephalopathy and their relationship to age and clinical features. AJNR Am *J Neuroradiol*. 2005;26(10):2481–2487.

Case 14

Please refer to the following images to answer the next three questions:

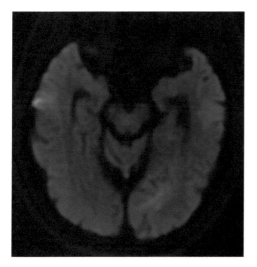

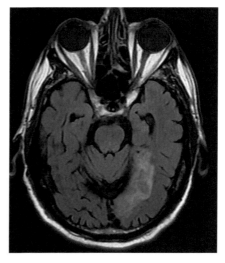

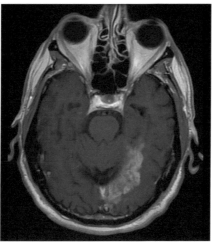

A 74-year-old male presents with two weeks of headache, dizziness, and memory problems.

14.1 What is the **MOST** likely diagnosis?

A. Glioblastoma.

B. Meningioma.

C. Metastasis.

D. Tumefactive demyelination.

E. Subacute infarct.

14.2 What is the **MOST** appropriate next step in management?

A. Biopsy.

B. Surgical resection.

C. Lumbar puncture.

D. CT of the chest, abdomen, and pelvis.

E. Follow-up MRI in 6 to 8 weeks.

14.3 What is the underlying pathophysiology resulting in enhancement of subacute infarcts?

A. Bloodbrain barrier breakdown.

B. Microglial activation.

C. Cytotoxic edema.

D. Increased deoxyhemoglobin fraction.

E. Luxury perfusion.

Answers and Explanations

14.1 Correct: E. Subacute infarct.

The images show cortical and subcortical T2 fluid-attenuated inversion recovery (FLAIR) signal abnormality in the left mesial temporal and occipital lobes, with intense gyral enhancement and mild diffusion signal. This abnormality follows the left posterior cerebral artery (PCA) vascular territory without surrounding vasogenic edema. These imaging findings are most consistent with a subacute PCA infarct, which fits the clinical picture of an acute onset of neurological symptoms two weeks prior to the MRI. Subacute infarcts can be aggressive appearing on imaging due to the presence of intense enhancement and may mimic a tumor. However, conformity to a vascular territory without surrounding reactive edema favors infarct as the top differential consideration.

Other choices and discussion
A. Glioblastoma is an aggressive primary brain neoplasm that often shows intense enhancement, although the radiographic appearance and enhancement are quite variable. Glioblastomas often have significant mass effect and surrounding vasogenic edema as well as cystic/necrotic portions and hemorrhage.
B. Meningiomas are extra-axial tumors which are usually intensely enhance. Determining the location of a lesion is often helpful, as the above case of enhancement is not only clearly intra-axial but the meningiomas are also extra-axial.
C. A metastasis can have a variable appearance but is often rounded in morphology and nearly always enhances. Surrounding vasogenic edema is common, especially with larger metastases.
D. Tumefactive demyelination is an inflammatory tumor mimic which may be quite large and have an aggressive appearance with enhancement, edema, and mass effect. However, tumefactive lesions often show a characteristic "leading edge" of peripheral or incomplete enhancement or diffusion signal along the lesion margin.

14.2 Correct: E. Follow-up MRI in 6 to 8 weeks.

Infarcts begin to show enhancement at 3 to 7 days after the onset and resolves after 4 to 6 weeks. Intense enhancement is expected in the subacute phase from 1 to 3 weeks. Obtaining a short-term follow-up MRI in 6 to 8 weeks can confirm the diagnosis of infarct, as enhancement associated with a subacute infarct is expected to resolve over time and volume loss starts to become apparent. In addition, a working diagnosis of subacute infarct should prompt a neurology consultation and a stroke workup.

Other choices and discussion
A and **B.** Biopsy and surgical resection would be considerations if tumor is the primary diagnostic consideration.
C. Lumbar puncture would be helpful when infection or inflammation/demyelination is suspected.
D. CT of the chest, abdomen, and pelvis should be obtained if cerebral metastases are suspected to find a primary malignancy.

14.3 Correct: A. Bloodbrain barrier breakdown.

Parenchymal enhancement in infracts, as well as enhancement in general, is due to breakdown of the bloodbrain barrier in the injured brain. As such enhancement is a nonspecific finding that is observed in many disorders including stroke, infection, demyelination, tumors, hemorrhage, and radiation necrosis. It is important to keep a broad differential in mind when encountering abnormal enhancement and use enhancement patterns (while taking the entire radiologic and clinical picture into consideration) to develop an appropriate differential diagnosis in a given case.

Other choices and discussion
B. Microglial activation occurs during stroke but cannot be directly imaged by today's standard MRI.
C. Cytotoxic edema is one of the first imaging manifestations in stroke and is represented by nonenhancing T2 signal and swelling in infarcted brain tissue in the acute phase.
D. The veins draining hypoperfused brain will demonstrate an increased deoxyhemoglobin fraction as the stressed tissue extracts more oxygen than in normal conditions. This manifests as increased susceptibility on gradient echo (GRE) or susceptibility-weighted imaging (SWI) images within these veins.
E. Luxury perfusion is hyperperfusion to infarcted brain after reperfusion and is independent of enhancement characteristics.

References

Karonen JO, Partanen PL, Vanninen RL, et al. Evolution of MR contrast enhancement patterns during the first week after acute ischemic stroke. AJNR *Am J Neuroradiol.* 2001;22(1): 103–111.

Smirniotopoulos JG, Murphy FM, Rushing EJ, et al. Patterns of contrast enhancement in the brain and meninges. *Radiographics.* 2007;27(2):525–551.

Case 15

Please refer to the following images to answer the next three questions:

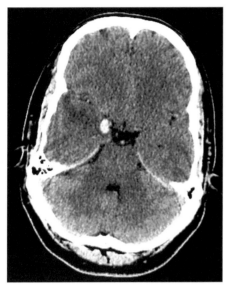

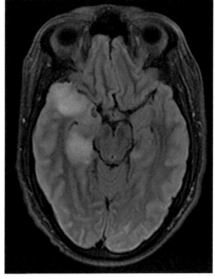

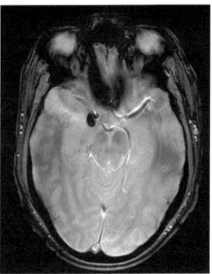

A 30-year-old male presents with one week of progressive headache and fever.

15.1 What is the **BEST** next step in diagnosis?

A. Computed tomography angiography (CTA) or magnetic resonance angiography (MRA).
B. Anticoagulation.
C. Lumbar puncture.
D. Biopsy.
E. Electroencephalogram (EEG).

15.2 What is the **MOST** likely diagnosis?

A. Ruptured aneurysm.
B. Venous thrombosis and hemorrhagic infarct.
C. Herpes encephalitis.
D. Glioma.
E. Seizure-related changes.

15.3 What imaging feature, if present, is helpful in distinguishing herpes encephalitis from autoimmune limbic encephalitis?

A. Temporal lobe involvement.
B. Hemorrhage.
C. Enhancement.
D. Cortical swelling.
E. Hyperperfusion.

Answers and Explanations

15.1 Correct: C. Lumbar puncture.

The computed tomography images show hypodensity and focal hemorrhage in the right temporal lobe. This is confirmed on magnetic resonance imaging with cortical swelling, T2 hyperintensity, and focal hemorrhage in the right temporal lobe as well as mild involvement of the left temporal lobe. Given acute onset and fever, the primary concern is infectious encephalitis, and thus, a lumbar puncture should be performed.

Other choices and discussion
A. Noninvasive vascular imaging with CTA or MRA would be performed to assess for aneurysm or arteriovenous malformation (AVM). An aneurysm in this location would typically bleed into the subarachnoid space (rather than be located in the parenchyma as in this case). AVM rupture is typically intraparenchymal; however, the focal hemorrhage shown is too small to account for the surrounding signal abnormality and does not account for the signal abnormality in the left temporal lobe.
B. Anticoagulation is the treatment of choice for venous infarcts.
D. Biopsy would be indicated if neoplasm is the primary concern.
E. An EEG is indicated if seizures are suspected.

15.2 Correct: C. Herpes encephalitis.

There is cortical swelling, T2 hyperintensity, and focal hemorrhage in the right temporal lobe, with mild involvement of the left temporal lobe. These are classic imaging findings of herpes encephalitis.

Other choices and discussion
A. Localizing the hemorrhage to the intra-axial space (brain parenchyma) is important, as the small hemorrhage in the uncus could be confused for extra-axial hemorrhage from a ruptured aneurysm.
B. Venous thrombosis and hemorrhagic infarct is a differential consideration for the right-sided findings, but the contralateral temporal involvement makes this much less likely than encephalitis.
D. Glioma can mimic encephalitis with cortical expansion, especially if unilateral, but is less likely to present with acute symptoms and fever.
E. Seizure-related changes may result in cortical edema and restricted diffusion; however, swelling is not a prominent feature and hemorrhage is not typically observed.

15.3 Correct: B. Hemorrhage.

Hemorrhage is rare in autoimmune encephalitis but common in herpes encephalitis, and thus useful in excluding an autoimmune etiology when present.

Other choices and discussion
A and **C–E.** Herpes encephalitis and autoimmune limbic encephalitis have overlapping imaging features, as both may involve the bilateral temporal lobes, with enhancement, cortical swelling, and hyperperfusion.

References

Noguchi T, Mihara F, Yoshiura T, et al. MR imaging of human herpesvirus-6 encephalopathy after hematopoietic stem cell transplantation in adults. *AJNR Am J Neuroradiol.* 2006;27(10):2191–2195.

Noguchi T, Yoshiura T, Hiwatashi A, et al. CT and MRI findings of human herpesvirus 6-associated encephalopathy: comparison with findings of herpes simplex virus encephalitis. AJR *Am J Roentgenol.* 2010;194(3):754–760.

Case 16

Please refer to the following images to answer the next three questions:

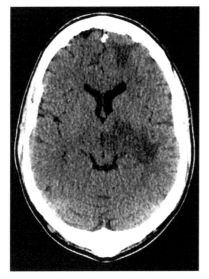

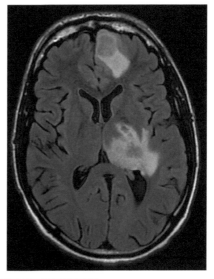

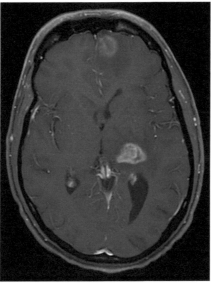

A 31-year-old male with history of HIV off treatment presents with altered mental status and right-sided weakness.

16.1 What is the **MOST** likely diagnosis?

A. Lymphoma.

B. Progressive multifocal leukoencephalopathy (PML).

C. HIV encephalitis.

D. Immune reconstitution inflammatory syndrome (IRIS).

E. Toxoplasmosis.

16.2 What imaging feature, if present, can help to distinguish between toxoplasmosis and lymphoma?

A. Diffusion restriction.

B. Hemorrhage.

C. Enhancement.

D. Surrounding vasogenic edema.

E. T2 hypointensity.

16.3 What imaging test is useful to help distinguish toxoplasmosis from lymphoma?

A. Contrast-enhanced CT.

B. Cisternography.

C. F-fluorodeoxyglucose (FDG) positron emission tomography (PET).

D. Functional magnetic resonance imaging (fMRI).

E. Ioflupane single-photon emission computed tomography (SPECT).

Answers and Explanations

16.1 Correct: E. Toxoplasmosis.

Toxoplasmosis is the most common cause of an intracranial "lesion" in patients with AIDS. Typical imaging features are present in this case. Lesions usually involve the basal ganglia, thalamus, and corticomedullary junction, and multiple lesions are common. Lesions are hypodense on computed tomography with surrounding vasogenic edema. On magnetic resonance imaging (MRI), they are T2 isointense or hypointense and demonstrate irregular enhancement. A "target sign" is a relatively specific but insensitive finding, with irregular peripheral enhancement surrounding a round nodule.

Other choices and discussion

A. Lymphoma is the primary differential consideration and may be indistinguishable from toxoplasmosis on MRI. However, it is less common than toxoplasmosis and is often considered after empiric treatment for toxoplasmosis fails.
B. PML shows asymmetric white matter T2 hyperintensity in the cerebral hemispheres involving the subcortical white matter with minimal mass effect. Enhancement is usually absent, although it is usually mild if present.
C. HIV encephalitis or AIDSdementia complex shows diffuse symmetric cerebral volume loss and confluent white matter T2 signal abnormality without enhancement.
D. IRIS occurs after institution of highly active antiretroviral therapy, and is the result of immune reaction to an underlying infection. The imaging appearance is variable and depends on the specific infection.

16.2 Correct B. Hemorrhage.

Hemorrhage may occur in toxoplasmosis but is very uncommon in untreated lymphoma.

Other choices and discussion

A and **C, E.** Diffusion restriction, enhancement, surrounding vasogenic edema, and lesional T2 hypointensity are commonly seen in both toxoplasmosis and lymphoma.

16.3 Correct: C. F-fluorodeoxyglucose (FDG) positron emission tomography (PET).

Lymphoma is hypermetabolic and often FDG avid, while toxoplasmosis is frequently "cold" on FDG PET.

Other choices and discussion

A. Contrast-enhanced CT does not provide additional diagnostic information if a contrast-enhanced MRI has already been obtained.
B. There is no role for cisternography, which is useful for detecting CSF leaks.
D. fMRI does not play a role in distinguishing toxoplasmosis and lymphoma.
E. Ioflupane SPECT is useful in the diagnosis of Parkinson's disease.

References

Offiah CE, Turnbull IW. The imaging appearances of intracranial CNS infections in adult HIV and AIDS patients. Clin Radiol. 2006;61(5):393–401.

Smith AB, Smirniotopoulos JG, Rushing EJ. From the archives of the AFIP: central nervous system infections associated with human immunodeficiency virus infection: radiologic-pathologic correlation. Radiographics. 2008;28(7):2033–2058.

Please refer to the following images to answer the next three questions:

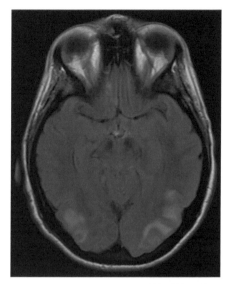
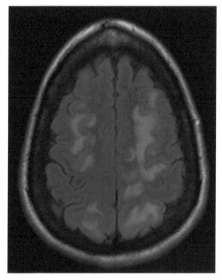
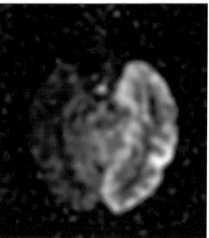

A 50-year-old male with history of hypertension presents with seizures.

17.1 What diagnosis accounts for the white matter signal abnormality on T2 fluid-attenuated inversion recovery (FLAIR) images?

A. Posterior reversible encephalopathy syndrome (PRES).
B. Progressive multifocal leukoencephalopathy (PML).
C. Creutzfeldt-Jakob disease (CJD).
D. Herpes simplex virus (HSV) encephalitis.
E. Gliomatosis cerebri.

17.2 What diagnosis accounts for the left-sided cerebral hyperperfusion on the arterial spin labeling (ASL) perfusion image?

A. Right internal carotid artery (ICA) stenosis.

B. Luxury perfusion after recanalization of left ICA occlusion.
C. Seizure activity.
D. Encephalitis.
E. Hypervascular tumor.

17.3 What MRI finding is associated with prolonged seizure activity?

A. Hippocampal edema and restricted diffusion.
B. "Cortical ribboning" with bilateral patchy cortical restricted diffusion.
C. Asymmetric bilateral temporal T2 signal abnormality and hemorrhage.
D. Restricted diffusion in the bilateral globi pallidi.
E. Selective volume loss in the caudate nuclei.

Answers and Explanations

17.1 Correct: A. Posterior reversible encephalopathy syndrome (PRES).

T2 FLAIR images show patchy signal hyperintensity in the subcortical white matter of both cerebral hemispheres with a posterior predominance, which is the classic imaging appearance of PRES. PRES is commonly associated with severe hypertension, eclampsia, and immunosuppressive medications, and is also thought to be related to loss of cerebrovascular autoregulation, resulting in vasodilation and edema. It is important to remember that PRES has variable imaging features beyond the typical presentation of parietaloccipital white matter involvement; these include the presence of bilateral asymmetric or unilateral cortical involvement, "central" brainstem and basal ganglia involvement, and hemorrhage.

Other choices and discussion

B. Progressive multifocal leukoencephalopathy (PML) is related to JC virus infection, which typically occurs in the setting of immunodeficiency. PML also involves the subcortical white matter including the subcortical U-fibers. Imaging features which can help in differentiating PML from PRES include greater asymmetry of signal abnormality and periventricular white matter involvement and, less commonly, cortical involvement. CJD is a neurodegenerative disease related to an abnormal prion isoform, with MRI showing restricted diffusion in the cortex and deep gray nuclei and progressive volume loss.
C, D. HSV encephalitis typically results in asymmetric expansile T2 signal in the mesial temporal lobes; hemorrhage is also common.
E. Gliomatosis cerebri describes an extensive growth pattern of infiltrative glioma and is no longer a distinct pathological entity according to the updated 2016 World Health Organization (WHO) classification. Infiltrative tumor results in marked cortical expansion and can also involve white matter.

17.2 Correct: C. Seizure activity.

Recent seizure activity can result in significant perfusion changes on ASL imaging, typically manifesting as high signal (hyperperfusion) to the affected cerebral cortex.

Other choices and discussion

A. Right-sided cerebral hypoperfusion from an ICA stenosis will manifest as asymmetry in cerebral perfusion; in this case, the left hemisphere has high signal and is abnormal. In practice, it may be necessary to assess the postprocessed quantitative or color cerebral blood flow (CBF) maps to determine the abnormal side.
B. Seizure activity does not have to conform to a vascular distribution, which is helpful in distinguishing this phenomenon from luxury perfusion-related to infarct-associated vascular occlusion and recanalization.
D. Perfusion findings in encephalitis are variable, and hyperperfusion may be present. However, no findings of encephalitis are present on the T2 FLAIR images to support this diagnosis.
E. Similarly, hypervascular tumors such as glioblastoma or meningioma may show hyperperfusion, but a mass-like lesion will be clearly present on the structural images.

17.3 Correct: A. Hippocampal edema and restricted diffusion.

Prolonged uncontrolled seizure activity or status epilepticus may result in excitotoxic damage to the hippocampus. This may manifest on MRI as cytotoxic edema with restricted diffusion and mildly expansile T2 signal in the hippocampus. If treated early, these finding are reversible, although they can result in hippocampal sclerosis chronically.

Other choices and discussion

B. "Cortical ribboning" with bilateral patchy cortical restricted diffusion describes classic findings of CJD.
C. Asymmetric bilateral temporal T2 signal abnormality and hemorrhage are findings of HSV encephalitis.
D. Restricted diffusion in the bilateral globi pallidi is a finding in hypoxia, specifically hypoxic injury related to carbon monoxide poisoning.
E. Selective volume loss in the caudate nuclei is characteristic of Huntington disease.

References

Shankar J, Banfield J. Posterior Reversible Encephalopathy Syndrome: A Review. Can Assoc *Radiol J.* 2017;68(2): 147–153.

Tranvinh E, Lanzman B, Provenzale J, et al. Imaging Evaluation of the Adult Presenting With New-Onset Seizure. *AJR Am J Roentgenol.* 2019;212(1):15–25.

Case 18

Please refer to the following images to answer the next three questions:

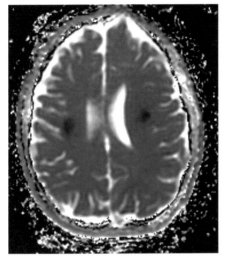

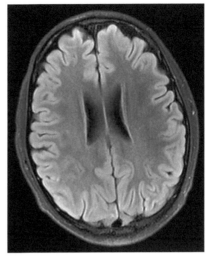

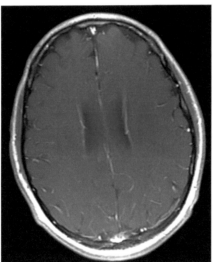

An 18-year-old male with history of lymphoma treated with intrathecal chemotherapy presents with altered mental status.

18.1 What is the **MOST** likely diagnosis?

A. Posterior reversible encephalopathy syndrome (PRES).

B. Methotrexate leukoencephalopathy.

C. Central nervous system (CNS) lymphoma.

D. Progressive multifocal leukoencephalopathy (PML).

E. Acute embolic infarcts.

18.2 What is the **BEST** next step in management?

A. Blood pressure management.

B. Brain biopsy.

C. Assess chemotherapy regimen.

D. MRA of the head and neck.

E. CSF PCR for JC virus.

18.3 What is the **MOST** common site of involvement of methotrexate leukoencephalopathy?

A. Centrum semiovale.

B. Subcortical U-fibers.

C. Corpus callosum.

D. Basal ganglia.

E. Brainstem.

Answers and Explanations

18.1 Correct: B. Methotrexate leukoencephalopathy.

Early MRI changes of methotrexate leukoencephalopathy are characterized by patchy restricted diffusion in the white matter, typically involving the centrum semiovale. There is no enhancement or mass effect. Early in the disease process, there is little to no T2 signal abnormality, although this may develop in the subsequent weeks.

Other choices and discussion

A. PRES typically demonstrates patchy T2 signal abnormality in the posterior cerebral subcortical and deep white matter, usually in the setting of hypertension. Enhancement may be present, and diffusion restriction is typically absent.

C. Parenchymal CNS involvement of lymphoma will show restricted diffusion due to the dense cellularity of the tumor as well as T2 signal abnormality and enhancement.

D. PML occurs due to latent JC virus infection in immunocompromised patients. MRI typically shows multiple areas of patchy T2 signal in the supratentorial white matter, classically involving the subcortical U-fibers, without enhancement or mass effect. Diffusion restriction may be present but is usually mild and at the periphery or "leading edge" of the lesion.

E. Acute embolic infarcts would also show restricted diffusion without enhancement or T2 signal; however, these are more common at the gray-white matter junction, and are more discrete compared with the patchy lesions in methotrexate leukoencephalopathy.

18.2 Correct: C. Assess chemotherapy regimen.

Diffusion-weighted imaging (DWI) changes in early methotrexate neurotoxicity are important to identify, and will help guide whether methotrexate should be held or adjunctive medications should be given.

Other choices and discussion

A. Managing elevated blood pressure is important in treating PRES.

B. Brain biopsy is an important but invasive procedure for assessing unknown brain lesions and suspected tumors, and would not be indicated in a clear case of methotrexate neurotoxicity.

D. MRA of the head and neck would be appropriate if acute stroke was suspected to assess the arterial vasculature.

E. Cerebrospinal fluid (CSF) polymerase chain reaction (PCR) for JC virus is obtained if PML is suspected.

18.3 Correct: A. Centrum semiovale.

Methotrexate leukoencephalopathy is a rare dose-dependent complication of methotrexate administration, which is often observed in children with leukemia.

Other choices and discussion

B. The earliest imaging manifestation is patchy diffusion restriction in the centrum semiovale, which may progress to confluent T2 signal abnormality involving the subcortical white and may involve the subcortical U-fibers.

C–E. The corpus callosum, basal ganglia, and brainstem are typically spared.

References

Fisher MJ, Khademian ZP, Simon EM et al. Diffusion-weighted MR imaging of early methotrexate-related neurotoxicity in children. *AJNR Am J Neuroradiol.* 2005;26:1686–1689.

Reddick WE, Glass JO, Helton KJ et al. Prevalence of leukoencephalopathy in children treated for acute lymphoblastic leukemia with high-dose methotrexate. *AJNR Am J Neuroradiol.* 2005;26(5):1263–1269.

Case 19

Please refer to the following images to answer the next three questions:

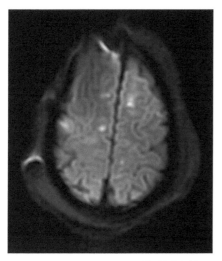

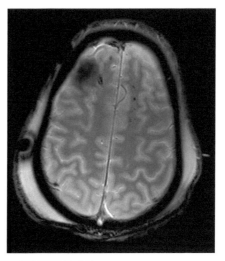

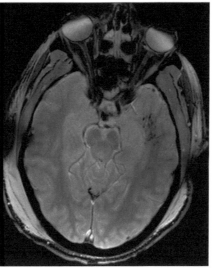

A 45-year-old male involved in a high-speed motor vehicle accident presents with a Glascow Coma Scale (GCS) score of 3.

19.1 What finding is demonstrated on diffusion- and susceptibility-weighted images (DWI and SWI, respectively)?

A. Fat emboli.

B. Cardiac thromboemboli.

C. Diffuse axonal injury.

D. Watershed hypoperfusion injury.

E. Cerebral vascular dysautoregulation.

19.2 What finding portends the most severe prognosis?

A. Concurrent subarachnoid hemorrhage.

B. Hydrocephalus.

C. Subcortical white matter involvement.

D. Corpus callosum involvement.

E. Brainstem involvement.

19.3 Which MRI sequence is most sensitive for detecting diffuse axonal injury?

A. T2-fluid-attenuated inversion recovery (FLAIR).

B. Susceptibility weighted imaging (SWIs).

C. Diffusion-weighted imaging (DWI).

D. T1 contrasted-enhanced imaging.

E. Arterial spin labeling (ASL) perfusion imaging.

Answers and Explanations

19.1 Correct: C. Diffuse axonal injury.

Diffuse axonal injury (DAI) is caused by axonal stretching or shearing, usually due to rapid deceleration in high-speed motor vehicle accidents. CT may be normal or show few small microhemorrhages. On MRI, DAI manifests as linear and ovoid foci of restricted diffusion and susceptibility in the affected white matter, oriented along the white matter tracts. The most common sites of involvement are the subcortical white matter, particularly at the gray–white matter junction in the paramedian frontal lobes and the corpus callosum. The basal ganglia and brainstem may also be involved.

Other choices and discussion

A. Fat emboli are another potential complication of trauma, and is the result of long bone fracture. Imaging findings of fat emboli syndrome overlap with DAI with multiple punctate foci of restricted diffusion on DWI; however, these typically occur in the watershed distribution or more diffusely than in DAI. In addition, in fat emboli, SWI demonstrates extensive tiny hemorrhages. In patients with high-speed trauma and long bone fractures, DAI and fat emboli may coexist.

B. Cardiac thromboemboli will show multiple small infarcts in one or multiple vascular territories, usually without hemorrhage.

D. Watershed hypoperfusion injury occurs during severe hypotension, especially if there is preexisting carotid or intracranial stenosis. MRI in hypoperfusion injury demonstrates multiple infarcts in the deep anterior cerebral artery-middle cerebral artery (ACA-MCA) and/or middle cerebral artery-posterior cerebral artery (MCA-PCA) watershed territories.

E. Cerebral vascular dysautoregulation is a contributing factor in posttraumatic cerebral edema, and does not result in discrete infarcts or hemorrhages.

19.2 Correct: E. Brainstem involvement.

DAI is graded by the Adams and Gennarelli staging criteria: Grade 3, or brainstem involvement, carries the highest morbidity and mortality. Grade 3 comprised of grade 2 lesions with brainstem involvement.

Other choices and discussion

C and D. defined by involvement of the gray-white junction and subcortical white matter; grade 2 is comprised of grade 1 lesions with corpus callosum involvement.

A and B. Concurrent subarachnoid hemorrhage and hydrocephalus are important complications to identify in trauma, but are not as severe as DAI with brainstem involvement.

19.3 Correct: C. Diffusion-weighted imaging (DWI).

DWI is the most sensitive modality to assess axonal injury.

Other choices and discussion

B. SWI is also very important in diffuse axonal injury (DAI) and may show multiple linear microhemorrhages, but in DAI they are less prevalent than DWI abnormalities, occurring in only 10 to 30% of cases. If hemorrhages predominate, it may indicate the patient has sustained a more severe diffuse vascular injury.

A. T2-FLAIR may show signal abnormality but is less sensitive than DWI.

D and E. T1 contrasted-enhanced images and ASL perfusion imaging do not have specific or sensitive findings in DAI.

References

Altmeyer W, Steven A, Gutierrez J. Use of Magnetic Resonance in the Evaluation of Cranial Trauma. *Magn Reson Imaging Clin N Am.* 2016;24(2):305–23.

Paterakis K, Karantanas AH, Komnos A, et al. Outcome of patients with diffuse axonal injury: the significance and prognostic value of MRI in the acute phase. *J Trauma.* 2000; 49:1071–1075.

Chapter 2 "Primary Effects of CNS Trauma" In: Anne G. Osborn, MD. Osborn's Brain: imaging, pathology, and anatomy. Second edition. [2nd ed.]

Case 20

Please refer to the following images to answer the next three questions:

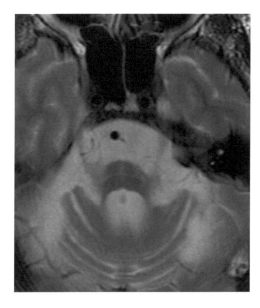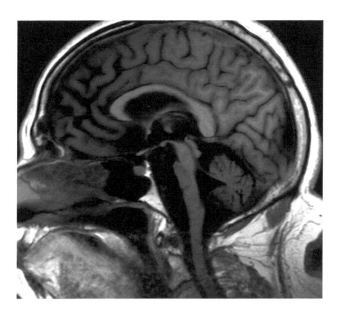

A 63-year-old female with cognitive difficulties and ataxia.

20.1 What is the **MOST** likely diagnosis?

A. Parkinson's disease.

B. Progressive supranuclear palsy.

C. Multiple system atrophy-cerebellar variant (MSA-c).

D. Spinocerebellar ataxia.

E. Huntington's disease.

20.2 What characteristic imaging finding is present?

A. Hot cross bun sign.

B. Swallow tail sign.

C. Hummingbird sign.

D. Molar tooth sign.

E. Empty delta sign.

20.3 What is the characteristic imaging finding of multiple system atrophy-Parkinsonian variant (MSA-p)?

A. Atrophy of the caudate nuclei.

B. Cortical ribboning on diffusion-weighted imaging (DWI).

C. Unilateral enlargement of the inferior olivary nucleus.

D. Bilateral anterior thalamic restricted diffusion.

E. Putaminal rim sign.

Answers and Explanations

20.1 Correct: C. Multiple system atrophy-cerebellar variant (MSA-c).

MSA-c is a progressive neurodegenerative disease characterized by cerebellar ataxia and autonomic failure. Parkinsonian features may also be present; if Parkinsonism is more pronounced than cerebellar features, it is classified as the Parkinsonian subtype (MSA-p). MRI plays an important role in diagnosis, as MSA-c is characterized by typical imaging features observed in this case, with cruciform T2 hyperintensity in the pons ("hot cross bun sign") and pontine and cerebellar atrophy.

Other choices and discussion

A. These findings are not present in Parkinson's disease, which can have an overlapping clinical presentation.
B. Progressive supranuclear palsy, another neurodegenerative syndrome, is characterized on imaging by midbrain volume loss rather than pontocerebellar atrophy.
D. Spinocerebellar ataxia is a heterogenous group of genetic disorders, in which similar findings to MSA-c have been reported in some variants; however, the onset is usually younger and the "hot cross bun sign" is less specific.
E. Huntington's disease results in severe caudate atrophy in the background of progressive global volume loss.

20.2 Correct: A. Hot cross bun sign.

The "hot cross bun" sign is a cruciform T2 hyperintensity in the pons related to intrinsic pontine atrophy, with preservation of the pyramidal tracts and pontine tegmentum. It was first associated with and is most specific for MSA-c; however, it has also been reported in a variety of conditions such as variant Creutzfeldt-Jakob disease, variants of spinocerebellar ataxia, and bilateral pontine infarction.

Other choices and discussion

B. Swallow tail sign, which is defined by a loss of the normal hyperintensity on SWI within Nigrosome-1 in the midbrain, is associated with Parkinson's disease.

C. The hummingbird sign refers to a diminutive appearance of the midbrain on sagittal images in progressive supranuclear palsy with midbrain atrophy.
D. The molar tooth sign refers to an elongated appearance of the superior cerebellar peduncles on axial images in Joubert syndrome.
E. Empty delta sign is observed in venous sinus thrombosis on contrasted-enhanced MRI or CT with a triangular filling defect in the venous sinus.

20.3 Correct: E. Putaminal rim sign.

The putaminal rim sign refers to T2 hyperintense signal between the lateral margin of the putamen and the external capsule due to volume loss and gliosis. It is only specific for MSA-p at 1.5 Tesla, and may be seen normally at 3 Tesla.

Other choices and discussion

A. Atrophy of the caudate nuclei is seen in Huntington's disease.
B. Cortical ribboning on DWI is characteristic of Creutzfeldt-Jakob disease.
C. Unilateral enlargement of the inferior olivary nucleus is observed in hypertrophic olivary degeneration.
D. Bilateral anterior thalamic restricted diffusion is most concerning for artery of Percheron infarct.

References

Fanciulli A, Wenning GK. Multiple-system atrophy. *N Engl J Med*. 2015;372(3):249–63.

Kim HJ, Jeon B, Fung VSC. Role of Magnetic Resonance Imaging in the Diagnosis of Multiple System Atrophy. *Mov Disord Clin Pract*. 2017;4(1):12–20.

Case 21

Please refer to the following images to answer the next three questions:

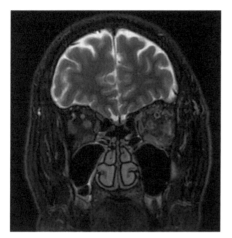

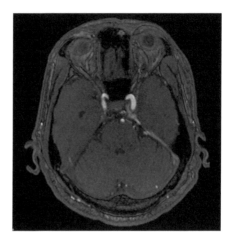

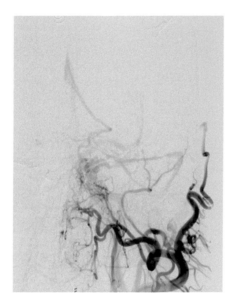

A 57-year-old male presents with three weeks of increasing redness in his left eye as well as increased intraocular pressure on ophthalmologic examination.

21.1 What is the cause of the eye redness and increased intraocular pressure?

A. Endophthalmitis.

B. Glaucoma.

C. Intraorbital venous hypertension.

D. Orbital mass.

E. Orbital pseudotumor.

21.2 What is the **MOST** likely diagnosis?

A. Orbital hemangioma.

B. Aneurysm of the cavernous internal carotid artery.

C. Developmental venous anomaly.

D. Indirect carotid-cavernous fistula (CCF).

E. Tolosa-Hunt syndrome.

21.3 What will MRI-based arterial spin labeling (ASL) perfusion imaging show in cases of carotid-cavernous fistulae (CCF)?

A. High signal in the cavernous sinus and surrounding veins.

B. Low signal in the cavernous internal carotid artery.

C. Hypoperfusion within the cerebral cortex ipsilateral to the fistula.

D. Hyperperfusion in the cerebral cortex in a non-vascular distribution.

E. Global cerebral hyperperfusion.

Answers and Explanations

21.1   Correct: C. Intraorbital venous hypertension.

High pressure in the cavernous sinus is transmitted to the orbit with conspicuous enlargement of the superior ophthalmic vein. This causes a measured increase in intraocular pressure and is responsible for the patient's symptoms.

Other choices and discussion
A. Endophthalmitis, an infection involving the globe, may also cause redness and increased intraocular pressure, but imaging would show irregular enhancement of the globe without the vascular findings in this case.
B. Glaucoma does not have specific CT or MR imaging findings.
D. An orbital mass is not seen on the images.
E. Orbital pseudotumor, or idiopathic orbital inflammation, is a nonneoplastic, inflammatory disorder which typically presents with orbital pain and swelling. There are a variety of imaging appearances, including diffuse inflammatory changes, which mimic infection and solid mass-like enhancing lesions from which the name pseudotumor is derived.

21.2   Correct: D. Indirect carotid-cavernous fistula (CCF).

The imaging shows an indirect v , with multiple vessels surrounding and forming a direct connection with the wall of the cavernous sinus. The Barrow classification is a useful system for dividing the different types of CCFs. A direct CCF results directly from the cavernous segment of the internal carotid artery (Barrow type A) usually due to trauma or from rupture of a cavernous internal carotid aneurysm. Indirect CCFs are not supplied by the cavernous internal carotid directly but rather by branches of the internal carotid artery (Barrow type B), external carotid artery (Barrow type C), or from both of these arteries (Barrow type D).

Other choices and discussion
A. Orbital hemangiomas, which are slow flow vascular malformations, are the most common vascular lesions of the orbit. On imaging, orbital hemangiomas are well-circumscribed masses, which progressively fill on multiphase, postcontrast imaging.
B. An aneurysm of the cavernous internal carotid artery may result in a direct CCF (Barrow type A) if it ruptures.
C. Developmental venous anomalies are found in the brain parenchyma and are anomalous veins which drain normal brain. They have a classic "medusa" or "stellate" appearance.
E. Tolosa-Hunt syndrome is a subtype of idiopathic orbital inflammatory disorder and involves the cavernous sinus. It typically presents with eye pain and cranial nerve palsies related to the involved nerves. Mass-like thickening of the cavernous sinus can also be observed.

21.3   Correct: A. High signal in the cavernous sinus and surrounding veins.

ASL perfusion MRI is helpful for diagnosis in cases of suspected arteriovenous shunting, as in dural arteriovenous fistulae (dAVFs) and cerebral arteriovenous malformations (AVMs). ASL can demonstrate the presence of arterial spins in the venous system, which are not normally present. In the case of CCFs, the shunt will result in high-ASL signal in the cavernous sinus, as well as in the outflow structures of the high-pressure cavernous sinus such as the superior ophthalmic vein. After the lesion has been treated with endovascular embolization or open surgical repair, ASL can also be helpful in identifying any residual or recurrent fistula, which manifests as persistent venous ASL signal.

Other choices and discussion
B. Low signal in the cavernous internal carotid artery is not an expected finding of CCFs.
C. Hypoperfusion to the cerebral cortex ipsilateral to the fistula will occur if there is a significant stenosis or occlusion of the internal carotid artery and there is insufficient collateral flow from the circle of Willis.
D. Hyperperfusion in the cerebral cortex in a nonvascular distribution is observed in patients with seizure and migraines.
E. Global cerebral hyperperfusion is noticed in normal young patients as well as in patients with hypercarbia.

References

Barrow DL, Spector RH, Braun IF, et al. Classification and treatment of spontaneous carotid-cavernous sinus fistulas. *J Neurosurg.* 1985 62:248–256.

Ellis JA, Goldstein H, Connolly ES, et al. Carotid-cavernous fistulas. *Neurosurg Focus.* 2012;32(5):E9.

Case 22

Please refer to the following images to answer the next three questions:

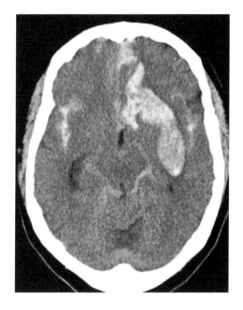 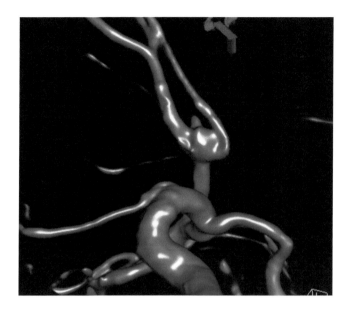

A 30-year-old male with no past medical history presents with altered mental status.

22.1 What is the etiology of the hemorrhage?

A. Dural arteriovenous fistula (dAVF).

B. Arteriovenous malformation (AVM).

C. Aneurysm.

D. Hypertensive emergency.

E. Cerebral amyloid angiopathy (CAA).

22.2 What is the **BEST** next step in management?

A. Conventional cerebral angiography.

B. Magnetic resonance imaging (MRI) with vessel wall imaging.

C. Lumbar puncture.

D. MRI with arterial spin labeling (ASL).

E. MR angiography.

22.3 What is the prognostic significance of an intra-parenchymal hematoma associated with ruptured aneurysms compared with aneurysmal subarachnoid hemorrhage alone?

A. Protective effect with improved patient outcomes.

B. Poorer outcomes with higher morbidity and mortality.

C. No effect on outcome.

D. Associated with risk of earlier rebleed.

E. Associated with a connective tissue disorder and higher risk of additional aneurysms.

Answers and Explanations

22.1 Correct: C. Aneurysm.

The large intraparenchymal hematoma in the inferior frontal lobes is immediately superior to an irregular outpouching of the left A1A2 junction of the left anterior cerebral artery (ACA) at the anterior communicating artery origin, as seen on the three-dimensional angiographic reconstructed image. This is a ruptured "A-comm aneurysm." While subarachnoid hemorrhage typically predominates after aneurysm rupture, an intraparenchymal hematoma may also be present. In fact, intraparenchymal hemorrhage may be the primary hemorrhage location if the aneurysm is closely associated with the cortex, such as in a superiorly directed A-comm aneurysm.

Other choices and discussion
A. dAVFs are acquired vascular lesions which result in a fistulous connection between an artery and dural venous sinus or cortical vein. The shunting can result in venous hypertension and intraparenchymal hemorrhage, with vascular imaging demonstrating enlarged arteries from external carotid artery branches associated with a venous sinus, and possibly enlarged cortical veins.
B. AVMs are congenital vascular lesions in an angiogenic nidus of abnormal arteriovenous connections without a capillary bed, and are a common and important cause of intraparenchymal hemorrhage. Vascular imaging will show a tangle of vessels around the nidus and enlarged feeding arteries and draining veins.
D. Hypertensive emergency may result in intraparenchymal hemorrhage due to small vessel rupture. While hypertension may "unmask" a preexisting aneurysm, typically no vascular abnormality is observed.
E. CAA may present with a lobar intraparenchymal hemorrhage without associated vascular lesion. MRI with gradient echo (GRE) or susceptibility-weighted images (SWI) may show numerous additional peripheral microhemorrhages.

22.2 Correct: A. Conventional cerebral angiography.

After the culprit ruptured aneurysm is identified by computed tomography angiography (CTA), a conventional or catheter digital subtraction angiogram, which has better spatial resolution and allows for finer and detailed assessment of the aneurysm and identification of small vessels

associated with the aneurysm prior to surgical clipping, is indicated. In addition, aneurysms that are amenable to endovascular coiling may be directly treated during the catheter angiogram.

Other choices and discussion
B. Vessel wall imaging on MRI may show enhancement of the inflamed aneurysm wall, but there is not sufficient evidence for this finding to direct treatment decisions.
C. Lumbar puncture is helpful in cases of suspected subarachnoid hemorrhage with a negative CT to test for xanthochromia and elevated red blood cells in cerebrospinal fluid (CSF).
D. MRI with ASL perfusion imaging is helpful in detecting shunting vascular lesions such as AVMs and dAVFs but does not typically aid in the diagnosis or characterization of aneurysms.
E. MR angiography is an alternative to CT angiography in the initial assessment of intracranial hemorrhage and also useful in aneurysm follow-up; however, it does not provide additional information acutely if a ruptured aneurysm is identified on CTA.

22.3 Correct: B. Poorer outcomes with higher morbidity and mortality.

Patients who have a ruptured aneurysm with an intraparenchymal hematoma tend to have higher mortality, and greater disability, if they survive, as compared with ruptured aneurysms with subarachnoid hemorrhage alone.

Other choices and discussion
A, C. An intraparenchymal hematoma associated with a ruptured aneurysm is associated with increased morbidity and mortality, not improved (**A**) or unaffected (**C**) outcomes.
D, E. There is not a significant correlation between the presence of intraparenchymal hematoma and earlier rebleeds (**D**) nor is there a clear association with connective tissue disorders (**E**).

References

Abbed KM, Ogilvy CS. Intracerebral hematoma from aneurysm rupture. *Neurosurg Focus*. 2003;15(4):E4.

Riina HA, Lemole GM Jr., Spetzler RF. Anterior communicating artery aneurysms. *Neurosurgery*. 2002;51:993–996.

Case 23

Please refer to the following images to answer the next three questions:

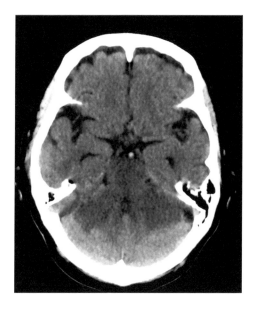

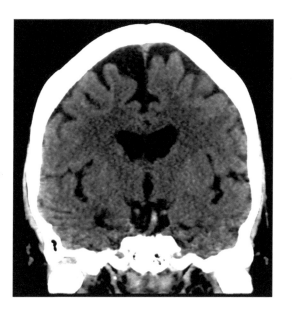

A 94-year-old female presents with decreased consciousness.

23.1 What sign is present?

A. Dense cerebellum sign.

B. Dense basilar sign.

C. Hummingbird sign.

D. Hot cross bun sign.

E. Molar tooth sign.

23.2 What is the best next step in diagnosis?

A. Computed tomography angiography/computed tomography perfusion (CTA/CTP).

B. Genetic testing.

C. Lumbar puncture.

D. MRI of the spine.

E. CT of the chest, abdomen, and pelvis.

23.3 What clinical syndrome is associated with basilar thrombosis?

A. Right arm and facial weakness and aphasia.

B. Homonymous hemianopsia.

C. Hemiballismus.

D. Crossed motor weakness (left facial and right extremity weakness).

E. Left lower extremity weakness.

Basilar Artery Thrombosis

Answers and Explanations

23.1 Correct: B. Dense basilar sign.

The "dense basilar sign," which is defined as increased density of the basilar artery on CT due to high-density clot, is seen with basilar artery occlusions caused by thromboembolism or in situ basilar artery thrombosis. It is important to specifically look for this sign as clinical symptoms of basilar artery occlusion are variable and may not be suspected clinically.

Other choices and discussion
A. The dense or white cerebellum sign is relative hyperdensity of the cerebellum compared to the cerebral parenchyma due to global cerebral hypoxic ischemia and cytotoxic edema.
C. The hummingbird sign describes the sagittal midline appearance of the midbrain and pons on CT or MRI in progressive supranuclear palsy, which results in midbrain atrophy.
D. The hot cross bun sign is an MRI finding in multiple system atrophy-cerebellar subtype, with pontine volume loss and a crossed-shaped hyperintensity in the midpons on T2-weighted images.
E. The molar tooth sign describes the elongated appearance of the superior cerebellar peduncles in Joubert syndrome.

23.2 Correct: A. Computed tomography angiography/computed tomography perfusion (CTA/CTP).

CT angiography allows for the assessment of the cerebral vasculature and delineation of the occlusion, while CT perfusion determines the core infarct and identifies if there is tissue at risk. With this information, it can be rapidly determined if the patient is a candidate for endovascular therapy to remove or lyse the clot.

Other choices and discussion
D. MRI of the brain (and not of the spine) with MR angiography and perfusion would also be useful; while it takes slightly longer to obtain, it provides more accurate determination of the core infarct.
B, C, and **E.** The other choices have no role in the initial assessment of basilar occlusion.

Note: The choice of CTA/CTP or MRI/MRP is often institution dependent, and more research is required to determine which one the superior technique.

23.3 Correct: D. Crossed motor weakness (left facial and right extremity weakness).

Basilar artery occlusion has variable presentation among different patients. Patients may present with nonfocal symptoms such as altered mental status, vertigo, or dysmetria from cerebellar or vestibular hypoperfusion, significant motor or sensory deficits, or, even rarely, locked-in syndrome. Crossed motor weakness, such as left facial weakness with right extremity weakness, results from hypoperfusion or ischemia to decussated ipsilateral motor fibers to the face and the nondecussated traversing corticospinal tract to the contralateral limb.

Other choices and discussion
A. Right arm and facial weakness and aphasia define the "left MCA syndrome," which is due to hypoperfusion to the important language areas in the left cerebral hemisphere and motor cortex supplied by the left middle cerebral artery.
B. Homonymous hemianopsia is visual field loss in both eyes to one side of midline and may be due to injuries to the optic pathway (from the optic tract to the primary visual cortex). Posterior cerebral artery (PCA) infarcts commonly present with homonymous hemianopsia.
C. Hemiballismus is a stereotyped unilateral choreiform movement disorder that results from an injury such as stroke or nonketotic hyperglycemia to the basal ganglia.
E. Left lower extremity weakness is observed with anterior cerebral artery occlusions, with hypoperfusion to the medial motor cortex, which controls the lower extremity.

References

Mortimer AM, Saunders T, Cook JL. Cross-sectional imaging for diagnosis and clinical outcome prediction of acute basilar artery thrombosis. *Clin Radiol.* 2011;66(6):551–558.

Ortiz de Mendivil A, Alcala-Galiano A, Ochoa M, et al. Brainstem stroke: anatomy, clinical and radiological findings. *Semin Ultrasound CT MR.* 2013;34:131–141.

Please refer to the following images to answer the next three questions:

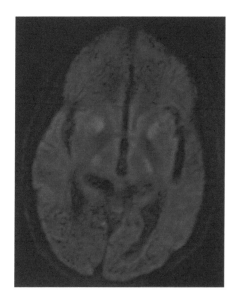 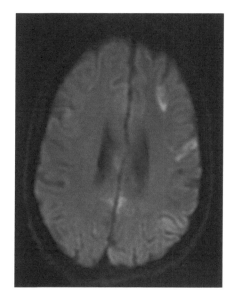

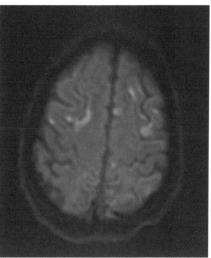

A 22-year-old female with prior history of stroke presents with new left-sided weakness.

24.1 What is the underlying cause of the multiple areas of restricted diffusion?

A. Cardiac thromboembolism.

B. Seizure activity.

C. Impaired cellular energy production.

D. Abnormal prion isoform.

E. Anterior circulation stenoocclusive disease (Moyamoya disease).

24.2 What test will confirm the diagnosis?

A. Gene sequencing.

B. Cerebrospinal fluid (CSF) testing for real-time quaking-induced conversion (RT-QuIC).

C. Electroencephalogram.

D. Conventional cerebral angiogram.

E. Echocardiogram.

24.3 What advanced MRI technique may improve specificity in diagnosis of mitochondrial encephalomyopathy, lactic acidosis, and stroke-like episodes (MELAS)?

A. Arterial spin labeling (ASL).

B. Dynamic contrast enhancement (DCE) MR perfusion.

C. Diffusion tensor imaging (DTI).

D. Functional MRI.

E. MR spectroscopy (MRS).

Answers and Explanations

24.1 Correct: C. Impaired cellular energy production.

The diffusion-weighted imaging (DWI) shows multiple areas of restricted diffusion in the cerebral cortex and deep grey nuclei bilaterally, most concerning for a toxic or metabolic process. In a young patient with a prior history of "stroke," this would be most concerning for a mitochondrial disorder, specifically mitochondrial encephalomyopathy, lactic acidosis, and stroke-like episodes (MELAS). MELAS is one of the most frequent mitochondrial diseases and has many manifestations, commonly including stroke-like episodes, dementia, epilepsy, myopathy, recurrent headaches, and short stature. Stroke-like episodes occur due to impaired energy production by dysfunctional mitochondria in the end organ and endothelium which can result in hypoperfusion and ischemia.

A. Cardiac thromboembolism may also show small areas of restricted diffusion, but these are typically located in the peripheral watershed distribution when a shower of small emboli occurs. Larger emboli may occlude the proximal cerebral vasculature and result in large territorial infarcts.

B. Prolonged seizure activity may result in cortical restricted diffusion in the affected cortex, which is usually confluent and unilateral.

D. An abnormal prion isoform is the cause of Creutzfeldt-Jakob disease, which causes cortical restricted diffusion, the so-called "cortical ribboning" in the basal ganglia and thalamus. The imaging picture can be similar to this case; however, clinically, the patient typically presents in middle or old age and has rapidly progressive dementia.

E. Anterior circulation stenoocclusive disease (Moyamoya disease) may cause infarcts in the deep anterior cerebral artery (ACA) middle cerebral artery (MCA) watershed territories as well as large territorial infarcts in the affected regions.

24.2 Correct: A. Gene sequencing.

Mitochondrial sequencing can confirm a suspected diagnosis of MELAS. The most common mutation is m.3243A>G mutation in the MT-TL1 gene. The diagnosis may also be made clinically with supporting evidence including lactic acidemia in blood or cerebrospinal fluid (CSF), MRI findings, and ragged red fibers on muscle biopsy.

Other choices and discussion

B. CSF testing for RT-QuIC is specific for Creutzfeldt-Jakob disease.

C. Electroencephalography is used to detect seizure activity.

D. Conventional cerebral angiogram is the gold standard diagnostic technique in assessing the cerebral vasculature and is usually normal in MELAS.

E. Echocardiography can detect intracardiac thrombi when a central thromboembolic source is suspected.

24.3 Correct: E. MR spectroscopy (MRS).

MRS in patients with MELAS typically shows a lactate peak, even in unaffected brain and CSF. MELAS is a mitochondrial disorder which presents in childhood or young adulthood with stroke-like symptoms, headache, dementia, seizure, and myopathy. MRI plays an important role in diagnosis with areas of restricted diffusion in a nonvascular distribution accounting for the "stroke-like" episodes as well as encephalomalacia in regions of prior metabolic injury. MR spectroscopy can improve specificity by demonstrating a lactate peak in unaffected regions.

Other choices and discussion

A–D. The other answer choices have not been proven to improve diagnosis in MELAS.

References

Castillo M, Kwock L, Green C. MELAS syndrome: imaging and proton MR spectroscopic findings. *AJNR Am J Neuroradiol.* 1995;16(2):233–239.

El-Hattab AW, Adesina AM, Jones J, et al. MELAS syndrome: Clinical manifestations, pathogenesis, and treatment options. *Mol Genet Metab.* 2015;116(1-2):4–12.

Sheerin F, Pretorius PM, Briley D, et al. Differential diagnosis of restricted diffusion confined to the cerebral cortex. *Clin Radiol.* 2008;63(11):1245–1253.

Case 25

Please refer to the following images to answer the next three questions:

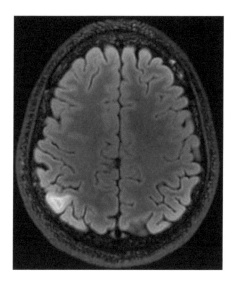
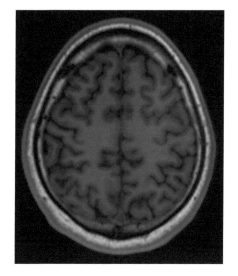

A 19-year-old male with a long-standing history of epilepsy and "abnormal MRI" as a baby presents for further evaluation.

25.1 What is the **MOST** likely diagnosis?

A. Cavernous malformation.

B. Heterotopic grey matter.

C. Focal cortical dysplasia.

D. Glioblastoma.

E. Ependymoma.

25.2 Which lobe is affected in the provided images?

A. Frontal.

B. Parietal.

C. Temporal.

D. Occipital.

E. Posterior fossa.

25.3 Which lobe is **MOST** sensitive to epileptogenic lesions?

A. Frontal.

B. Parietal.

C. Temporal.

D. Occipital.

E. Cerebellum.

Answers and Explanations

25.1 Correct: C. Focal cortical dysplasia.

The MR images show focal cortical thickening with linear T2/FLAIR signal abnormality in the adjacent white matter. This best describes focal cortical dysplasia (FCD), a congenital disorder of cortical malformation that is associated with epilepsy. Additional findings which are suggestive of FCD include blurring of the greywhite matter junction, abnormal gyration, and extension of T2 white matter signal to the ventricular margin ("transmantle sign"). A benign or indolent lesion is consistent with both the radiographic appearance and the report of an abnormality as a baby, although we cannot be certain this abnormality is the same and stable without direct comparison. Other differential considerations include gangliocytoma, ganglioglioma, and dysembryoplastic neuroepithelial tumor.

Other choices and discussion

A. Cavernous malformations are benign vascular lesions of abnormally dilated capillary vessels which are prone to rupture and hemorrhage. They are typically "bubbly" T2 hyperintense lesions with a peripheral hypointense rim due to hemosiderin staining from prior hemorrhage.
B. Heterotopic gray matter is a congenital lesion of neuronal migration, with gray matter in an abnormal location in the brain, most commonly along the ventricular margin. Heterotopic gray matter follows normal gray matter on all sequences and is not associated with T2 signal abnormality.
D and **E.** Aggressive neoplasms such as glioblastoma and ependymoma are unlikely in this case given the indolent clinical and radiographic course.

25.2 Correct: B. Parietal.

Determining which lobe contains a lesion can be difficult, especially on axial images if the angulation of the images is different from what is expected. However, one reliable method used to find the central sulcus on axial images is by identifying the superior frontal sulcus, which courses anteroposteriorly just lateral to the superior frontal gyrus. The superior frontal sulcus usually terminates posteriorly at the precentral sulcus, so the next sulcus posteriorly is the central sulcus. In this case, the T1 image shows the anteroposteriorly oriented superior frontal sulcus on the upper half of the image, ending in front of the hand knob of the central sulcus. The lesion is clearly posterior to the central sulcus and is, therefore, located in the parietal lobe.

Other choices and discussion

A. The lesion is not anterior to the central sulcus so, therefore, it is not in the frontal lobe.
C. The lateral fissure (Sylvian fissure) separates the temporal lobe from the frontal and parietal lobes. As the lesion is located above this fissure, it is not in the temporal lobe.
D. Differentiating the parietal and occipital lobes is best achieved on sagittal images by identifying the obliquely oriented parietooccipital sulcus. The lesion is not in the occipital lobe.
E. The lesion is located in the supratentorial brain; therefore, this answer choice is incorrect.

25.3 Correct: C. Temporal.

The temporal lobe is the most sensitive to developing seizures from brain lesions or other insults.

Other choices and discussion

A, B, D, E. Lesions in the frontal, parietal, and occipital lobes and cerebellum are less often epileptogenic, but the potential for seizure remains.

References

Colombo N, Salamon N, Raybaud C, et al. Imaging of malformations of cortical development. *Epileptic Disord.* 2009;11:194–205.

Colombo N, Tassi L, Galli C, et al. Focal cortical dysplasias: MR imaging, histopathologic, and clinical correlations in surgically treated patients with epilepsy. *AJNR Am J Neuroradiol.* 2003;24(4):724–733.

Case 26

Please refer to the following images to answer the next three questions:

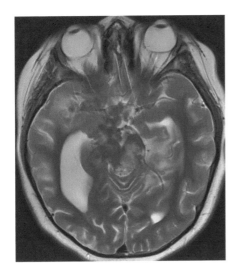 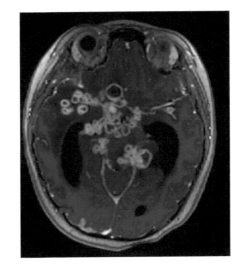

A 10-year-old female presents with progressive fever, chills, and irritability.

26.1 What is the **MOST** likely diagnosis?

A. Atypical or fungal infection.

B. Sarcoidosis.

C. Leptomeningeal carcinomatosis.

D. IgG4-related disease.

E. Viral meningitis.

26.2 What complication is evident on the images shown?

A. Hydrocephalus.

B. Cerebral infarction.

C. Transtentorial herniation.

D. Papilledema.

E. Hemorrhage.

26.3 Seeding of the meninges in tuberculous meningitis **MOST** commonly occurs via what method of spread?

A. Direct extension from calvarial infection.

B. Direct extension from mastoid infection.

C. Direct extension from sinus infection.

D. Hematogenous dissemination from distant source.

E. Retrograde neural spread.

Answers and Explanations

26.1   Correct: A. Atypical or fungal infection.

The axial T2-weighted and contrast-enhanced T1-weighted images show extensive enhancing material centered within the basal cisterns, with extension into the adjacent brain parenchyma. This material is T2 hypointense and solidly enhancing, with rim enhancement of the larger lesions. Taking into account the patient's young age and presence of a fever, atypical infection from mycobacterial and fungal microorganisms is the primary differential consideration. This patient is afflicted with tuberculous meningitis and cerebritis. Lumbar puncture with acid-fast staining and acid-fast bacteria (AFB) culture is warranted in addition to broader cerebrospinal fluid (CSF) analysis.

Other choices and discussion

B. Other granulomatous processes such as sarcoidosis are important but less likely differential considerations with basilar meningitis.
C. Leptomeningeal carcinomatosis, similarly, is less likely but important to consider. In the above case, the cystic foci, young age, and fever favor infection over tumor. Neoplasm should be reconsidered if the infectious workup is negative.
D. IgG4-related disease is a cause of hypertrophic pachymeningitis and not basal leptomeningitis.
E. Viral meningitis can cause thin leptomeningeal enhancement along the brain surfaces; it generally does not cause thick basilar meningitis and cerebritis.

26.2   Correct: A. Hydrocephalus.

The temporal horns of the lateral ventricles are significantly dilated and related to communicating hydrocephalus as a result of CSF obstruction in the basal cisterns. Hydrocephalus is the most common complication of tuberculous meningitis.

Other choices and discussion

B. Cerebral infarction is another common complication, resulting from arteritis of the vessels in the subarachnoid spaces by surrounding exudate with secondary thrombosis. In this case, edema related to parenchymal tuberculomas is present, but infarction is not demonstrated.
C. Transtentorial herniation can occur rarely as a result of severe hydrocephalus but is not observed here.
D. Papilledema may be evident on fundoscopic examination related to increased intracranial pressure; however, the degree of papilledema must be severe for it to be evident on MRI.
E. Hemorrhage is an uncommon complication and is not evident in this case.

26.3   Correct: D. Hematogenous dissemination from distant source.

Tuberculous meningitis is typically the result of hematogenous seeding from a distant source to the subpial brain. The subpial granuloma grows and ruptures into the subarachnoid space, and meningitis subsequently develops. This may occur during active TB infection elsewhere in the body, or the granuloma may lie quiescent for years after initial infection and seeding before reactivation. Once TB meningitis is diagnosed, workup of other sites of active infection should be pursued, especially pulmonary involvement.

Other choices and discussion

A–C. Direct extension from calvarial, mastoid, or sinus infection is a rare but potential source for TB meningitis, and these regions should be directly assessed on brain MRI for potential involvement.
E. While retrograde neural spread is a route of migration to the brain for some viruses such as Rabies and HSV1/2, it is not a recognized route for the spread of tuberculosis.

References

Bernaerts A, Vanhoenacker FM, Parizel PM, et al. Tuberculosis of the central nervous system: overview of neuroradiological findings. *Eur Radiol.* 2003;13(8):1876–1890.

Jinkins JR, Gupta R, Chang KH, et al. MR imaging of central nervous system tuberculosis. Radiol *Clin North Am.* 1995;33:771–786.

Case 27

Please refer to the following images to answer the next three questions:

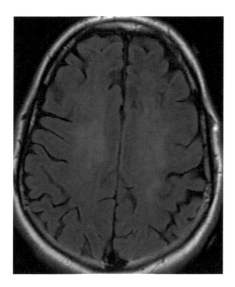

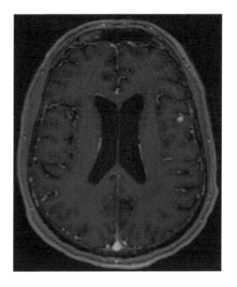

A 56-year-old HIV-positive male presents with altered mental status.

27.1 Which of the following statements regarding HIV encephalopathy is **TRUE**?

A. White matter lesions are uncommon.

B. Cognitive impairment is rare if there has been favorable response to highly active antiretroviral therapy (HAART).

C. Presents with symmetric basal ganglia calcifications in adults.

D. White matter lesions can involve the gray white matter junction.

E. Can present with seizures.

27.2 The second image demonstrates which of the following findings?

A. Parenchymal lesion.

B. Aneurysm.

C. Venous thrombus.

D. Subependymal enhancement.

E. Leptomeningeal enhancement.

27.3 Which of the following represents an atypical site for a mycotic aneurysm?

A. P3 PCA branch.

B. Petrous internal carotid artery.

C. Anterior communicating artery.

D. Calcarine artery.

E. Lateral frontobasal artery.

Answers and Explanations

27.1 Correct: D. White matter lesions can involve the gray-white matter junction.

HIV encephalopathy manifests as diffuse parenchymal volume loss and confluent T2 white matter lesions that can involve the subcortical U-fibers.

Other choices and discussion

A. Diffuse volume loss is related to direct neuronal damage from HIV infection; although not entirely clear, the white matter T2 signal changes are felt to be related to increased water retention.

B. Cognitive impairment is a major clinical manifestation of primary HIV encephalitis, commonly observed even in patients undergoing HAART.

C. In-utero HIV infection can manifest with symmetric basal ganglia calcification, which is not seen in cases of HIV infection acquired later in life.

E. Seizures are not caused by the primary HIV infection; if present, they are a red flag for underlying HIV-related malignancy and opportunistic infection.

27.2 Correct: B. Aneurysm.

The second, postcontrast T1-weighted image shows a focal aneurysmal sac along a left M3 MCA branch.

Other choices and discussion

A. This lesion is not located in the brain parenchyma.

C. This lesion does not involve a cortical vein.

D, E. Subependymal and leptomeningeal enhancement do not usually manifest on imaging as a focal round lesion. In addition, this lesion does not involve the ependyma (lining of the ventricles).

27.3 Correct: C. Anterior communicating artery.

Mycotic aneurysms, representing less than 5% of aneurysms, are associated with infection/inflammation. They are commonly observed in patients with HIV/AIDS, septicemia, infective endocarditis related to IV drug abuse, and increasingly in relatively immunocompromised states such as diabetes.

Other choices and discussion

A, D, E. The anterior communicating artery is one of the most common sites for an incidental saccular cerebral aneurysm. Mycotic aneurysms, however, are often irregular fusiform arterial outpouchings occurring at sites atypical for saccular cerebral aneurysms such as distal intracranial branch vessels.

B. The petrous segment of the internal carotid artery also represents an atypical location for a saccular aneurysm; hence, a mycotic aneurysm should be considered in the clinical setting of infection.

References

Allen LM, Fowler AM, Walker C, et al. Retrospective Review of Cerebral Mycotic Aneurysms in 26 Patients: Focus on Treatment in Strongly Immunocompromised Patients with a Brief Literature Review. *AJNR Am J Neuroradiol.* 2013;34(4):823–827.

Lee WK, Mossop PJ, Little AF, et al. Infected (Mycotic) Aneursyms: Spectrum of Imaging Appearances and Management. *Radiographics.* 2008;28(7):1853–1868.

Sailer AM, Wagemans BA, Nelemans PJ, et al. Diagnosing intracranial aneurysms with MR angiography: systematic review and meta-analysis. *Stroke.* 2014;45(1):119–126.

Case 28

Please refer to the following images to answer the next three questions:

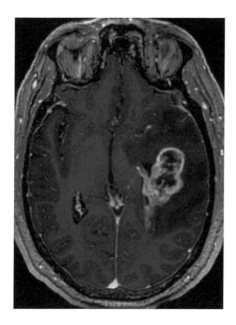

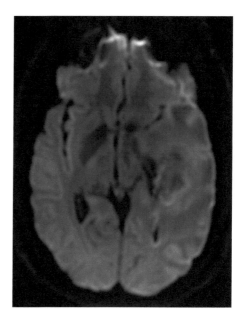

A 63-year-old male presenting with seizures.

28.1 What is the **MOST** likely diagnosis?

A. Pyogenic abscess.

B. Subacute infarct.

C. Lymphoma.

D. Glioblastoma.

E. Tumefactive multiple sclerosis.

28.2 Which additional feature is demonstrated by the provided images?

A. Satellite lesion.

B. Ventricular extension.

C. Obstructive hydrocephalus.

D. Venous sinus thrombosis.

E. Hemorrhage.

28.3 Which of the following combination of biomarkers and treatment provide the **MOST** favorable prognosis in glioblastoma?

A. IDH mutant, unmethylated MGMT promoter, resection, radiation.

B. IDH wild-type, methylated MGMT promoter, radiation, chemotherapy.

C. IDH wild-type, unmethylated MGMT promoter, resection, chemotherapy.

D. Unmethylated MGMT promoter, resection, radiation, chemotherapy.

E. IDH mutant, methylated MGMT promoter, resection, radiation.

Answers and Explanations

28.1 Correct: D. Glioblastoma.

Diffusion-weighted imaging (DWI) and postcontrast T1 images demonstrate a peripherally restricting and enhancing, centrally necrotic mass within the left temporal lobe, most consistent with a glioblastoma.

Other choices and discussion

A. Pyogenic abscess should demonstrate profound, central restricted diffusion.

B. Subacute infarct generally presents as nonmass-like enhancement without central necrosis.

C. In the absence of treatment, lymphoma generally does not demonstrate central necrosis and presents with a higher degree of restricted diffusion than glioblastoma.

E. Tumefactive multiple sclerosis presents with an incomplete ring of enhancement and diffusion restriction.

28.2 Correct: B. Ventricular extension.

The left temporal lobe mass extends into the body of the left lateral ventricle and abuts the choroid plexus, which predisposes to ventricular seeding of tumor.

Other choices and discussion

A, C, D. No evidence of satellite lesion, obstructive hydrocephalus, or venous sinus thrombosis is observed.

E. The provided images are not sufficient for the evaluation of hemorrhage, which would be better assessed on precontrast T1, T2* GRE, and SWI (susceptibility-weighted imaging).

28.3 Correct: E. IDH mutant, methylated MGMT promoter, resection, radiation.

Isocitrate dehydrogenase (IDH) gene mutations have been recognized as important genetic prognostic markers for diffuse gliomas and are now part of the latest WHO classification system of central nervous system (CNS) tumors (2016). In contrast to IDH wild-type glioblastomas, which are considered de novo and have a poorer prognosis, IDH mutant glioblastomas are thought to represent secondary tumors likely arising from a lower grade lesion. Given the answer choices, the last choice is most likely to have the best prognosis.

Other choices and discussion

A–D. IDH mutant-type glioblastomas with methylation of the MGMT promoter are more sensitive to treatment than IDH wild-type glioblastomas or those IDH mutant glioblastomas with an unmethylated MGMT promoter, and hence have the most favorable outcome. Maximal safe resection of the primary lesion followed by both chemotherapy and radiation has shown to prolong survival the most—more than resection, radiation, or chemotherapy alone. However, the fourth answer choice is eliminated since an unmethylated MGMT promoter confers relative treatment resistance, especially to temozolomide (chemotherapy).

References

Chen JR, Yao Y, Xu HZ, et al. Isocitrate Dehydrogenase (IDH)1/2 Mutations as Prognostic Markers in Patients With Glioblastomas. *Medicine (Baltimore)*. 2016;95(9): e2583.

Chen Y, Hu F, Zhou Y, et al. MGMT promoter methylation and glioblastoma prognosis: a systematic review and meta-analysis. *Arch Med Res*. 2013;44(4):281–290.

Louis DN, Perry A, Reifenberger, et al. The 2016 World Health Organization Classification of Tumors of the Central Nervous System: a summary. *Acta Neuropathol*. 2016;131(6):803–820.

Stupp R, Mason WP, van den Bent MJ, et al. Radiotherapy plus concomitant and adjuvant temozolomide for glioblastoma. *N Engl J Med*. 2005;352(10):987–996.

Case 29

Please refer to the following images to answer the next three questions:

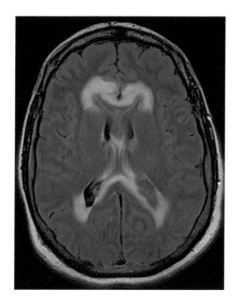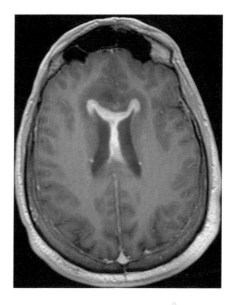

A 56-year-old male with altered mental status.

29.1 What is the **MOST** likely diagnosis in this immunocompetent patient?

A. High-grade glioma.

B. Neurosarcoidosis.

C. Lymphoma.

D. Progressive multifocal leukoencephalopathy.

E. Toxoplasmosis.

29.2 Which additional imaging sequence can support the diagnosis?

A. T2* gradient echo (T2* GRE).

B. Diffusion-weighted imaging (DWI).

C. Susceptibility-weighted imaging (SWI).

D. Noncontrast T1.

E. Single shot fast spin echo (T2 SSFSE).

29.3 Which of the following statements regarding primary CNS lymphoma is **FALSE**?

A. Hemorrhagic and necrotic lesions are common in immunocompromised patients.

B. Highly active antiretroviral therapy (HAART) has significantly reduced the occurrence of CNS lymphoma in AIDS patients.

C. Disease manifests later in life in immunocompetent patients compared to immunocompromised patients.

D. Treatment involves complete resection followed by chemotherapy and radiation.

E. Prognosis is generally better than glioblastoma.

Answers and Explanations

29.1 Correct: C. Lymphoma.

Postcontrast T1 image demonstrates homogenous subependymal/periventricular enhancement with involvement of the corpus callosum and surrounding T2 fluid-attenuated inversion recovery (FLAIR) abnormality. Findings are characteristic of primary central nervous system (CNS) lymphoma.

Other choices and discussion

A. Although high-grade gliomas can involve the corpus callosum, they often present with heterogenous enhancement and/or central necrosis in up to 95% of cases.
B. Leptomeningeal and dural involvement are more common than parenchymal involvement in neurosarcoidosis.
D. Progressive multifocal leukoencephalopathy is seen as confluent nonenhancing white matter T2 hyperintensity involving the subcortical U fibers in immunocompromised patients.
E. Toxoplasmosis is also observed in immunocompromised patients and classically presents as multiple enhancing target lesions without subependymal involvement.

29.2 Correct: B. Diffusion-weighted imaging (DWI).

Lymphoma tends to have characteristic diffusion restriction related to hypercellularity, with lower apparent diffusion coefficient (ADC) values than high-grade gliomas.

Other choices and discussion

A, C. T2 GRE and SWI can assess for underlying hemorrhage which is, however, not typically seen in immunocompetent or untreated patients.
D, E. These answer choices do not add any diagnostic value to this case.

29.3 Correct: D. Treatment involves complete resection followed by chemotherapy and radiation.

Option **D** is a false statement since the majority of CNS lymphoma lesions are very infiltrative and usually respond very well to chemotherapy. Lymphoma is confirmed on stereotactic biopsy and treated with chemotherapy with or without radiation. Given the great response to treatment, surgical resection is not typically necessary.

Other choices and discussion

A–C, E. Although CNS lymphoma has a poor prognosis, the prognosis is still better than glioblastoma, with a mean survival of 50 months in immunocompetent patients and 36 months in immunocompromised patients.

References

Ko CC, Tai MH, Li CF, et al. Differentiation between Glioblastoma Multiforme and Primary Cerebral Lymphoma: Additional Benefits of Quantitative Diffusion-Weighted MR Imaging. *PLoS ONE.* 2016;11(9):e0162565.

Mansour A, Qandeel M, Abdel-Razeq H, et al. MR imaging features of intracranial primary CNS lymphoma in immune competent patients. *Cancer Imaging.* 2014;14:22.

Osborn AG, Salzman KL, Jhaveri MD. *Diagnostic Imaging: Brain.* 3rd ed. Elsevier; 2016:566–569.

Toh CH, Castillo M, Wong AM, et al. Primary cerebral lymphoma and glioblastoma multiforme: differences in diffusion characteristics evaluated with diffusion tensor imaging. *AJNR Am J Neuroradiol.* 2008;29(3):471–475.

Case 30

Please refer to the following images to answer the next three questions:

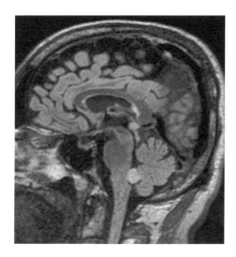

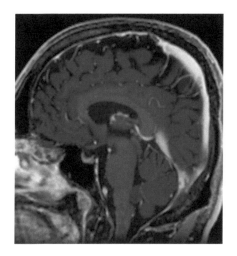

A 57-year-old male with memory issues.

30.1 What is the **MOST** likely diagnosis?

A. Meningioma.
B. Subependymoma.
C. Ependymoma.
D. Choroid plexus papilloma.
E. Metastasis.

30.2 What is the **BEST** next step in management?

A. Serial imaging.
B. Surgical resection.
C. Shunt placement.
D. Radiosurgery.
E. No intervention or follow-up.

30.3 Which of the following statements regarding ependymomas is **TRUE**?

A. The majority of ependymomas are supratentorial.
B. They are WHO grade I tumors.
C. They rarely demonstrate cerebrospinal (CSF) seeding.
D. They usually have low-signal on apparent diffusion coefficient (ADC).
E. The majority of supratentorial ependymomas are extraventricular.

Answers and Explanations

30.1 Correct: B. Subependymoma.

The provided images show a T2 fluid-attenuated inversion recovery (FLAIR) hyperintense, well-circumscribed, and nonenhancing lesion within the lower aspect of the fourth ventricle. The imaging findings and location are characteristic of a subependymoma.

Other choices and discussion
A, C–E. The remainder of the lesions should demonstrate contrast enhancement.

30.2 Correct: A. Serial imaging.

Subependymomas present in the middle-aged and elderly population and are frequently incidentally detected on imaging obtained for other reasons, as in this case. Most patients are asymptomatic; however, up to 30 to 40% of patients can become symptomatic, which can be related to increased intracranial pressure from obstructive hydrocephalus. Hence follow-up on serial imaging is generally recommended to assess for growth of the lesion and any signs of developing hydrocephalus.

Other choices and discussion
B. Surgical resection is curative but is usually not the first line of approach in management; resection is often reserved for symptomatic cases.
C. Shunt placement can be considered if hydrocephalus was present.
D. Radiosurgery is not a standard treatment for subependymomas.
E. As stated above, serial imaging is generally recommended to assess for lesion growth and signs of developing hydrocephalus.

30.3 Correct: E. The majority of supratentorial ependymomas are extraventricular.

About a third of all ependymomas are supratentorial, and the majority of those lesions tend to be extraventricular in location, arising from ependymal rests located along the ventricular margins.

Other choices and discussion
A. Only about a third of all ependymomas are supratentorial. The majority are infratentorial.
B. Ependymomas are either WHO grade II or III tumors depending on the histologic criteria. In contrast, myxopapillary ependymomas and subependymomas are benign WHO grade I tumors.
C. Up to 20% of ependymomas demonstrate CSF seeding and, therefore, imaging of the entire neuroaxis is warranted on initial diagnosis as well as at post-treatment surveillance timepoints.
D. Medulloblastomas and other primitive neuroectodermal tumors (PNET) demonstrate low signal on ADC (diffusion restriction), which is related to hypercellularity; ependymomas generally do not show diffusion restriction.

References

Bi Z, Ren X, Zhang J, et al. Clinical, radiological, and pathological features in 43 cases of intracranial subependymoma. *J Neurosurg.* 2015;122(1):49–60.

Niazi TN, Jensen EM, Jensen RL. WHO Grade II and II supratentorial hemispheric ependymomas in adults: case series and review of treatment options. *J Neurooncol.* 2009;91(3):323–328.

Case 31

Please refer to the following images to answer the next three questions:

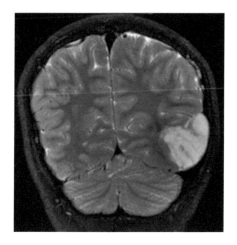 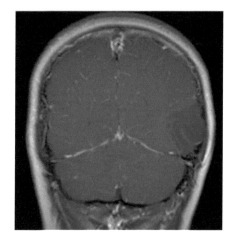

A 9-year-old male presents with treatment-resistant temporal lobe epilepsy.

31.1 What is the **MOST** likely diagnosis?

A. Glioblastoma.

B. Pleomorphic xanthoastrocytoma (PXA).

C. Ganglioglioma.

D. Dysembryoplastic neuroepithelial tumor (DNET).

E. Desmoplastic infantile ganglioglioma (DIG).

31.2 Which of the following statements regarding neuroepithelial neoplasms is **TRUE**?

A. DNET is the most common cause of tumor-related temporal lobe epilepsy.

B. The majority of these lesions arise from the subcortical white matter.

C. DNET is frequently associated with cortical dysplasia.

D. Most occur within the frontal lobe.

E. Ganglioglioma incidence peaks in the 30- to 40-year-old age group.

31.3 Which of the following entity **DOES NOT** present as a cyst containing a nodule on imaging?

A. Neurocysticercosis.

B. Ganglioglioma.

C. Pleomorphic xanthoastrocytoma (PXA).

D. Subependymal giant cell astrocytoma (SGCA).

E. Desmoplastic infantile astrocytoma (DIA).

Answers and Explanations

31.1 Correct: D. Dysembryoplastic neuroepithelial tumor (DNET).

The provided images show a mass-like T2 hyperintense and "bubbly" lesion involving the cortex of the posterior left temporal lobe with no enhancement. There is thinning of the overlying bone suggestive of a slow-growing lesion. Imaging findings are most consistent with DNET.

Other choices and discussion
A–C, E. The other lesions all typically demonstrate some degree of contrast enhancement. PXAs and gangliogliomas are also cortical-based lesions that frequently present as cysts with enhancing mural nodules. A dural tail is often seen in PXAs and 50% of gangliogliomas are calcified. DIG are large cystic tumors with enhancing mural nodules and the majority are seen in the infant population. Glioblastomas present as infiltrative and necrotic masses with nodular enhancement and are more common in older adults than in children.

31.2 Correct: C. DNET is frequently associated with cortical dysplasia.

Of the neuroepithelial tumors, DNETs are most commonly associated with focal cortical dysplasia.

Other choices and discussion
A, B, D, E. The remainder of the answer choices are incorrect. Gangliogliomas are the most common cause of tumor-related temporal lobe epilepsy. Neuroepithelial tumors arise from the cerebral cortex and not white matter. Most neuroepithelial tumors occur within the temporal lobes. Greater than 80% of gangliogliomas are seen in patients younger than 30 years of age with a peak incidence in the 10- to 20-year-old age group.

31.3 Correct: D. Subependymal giant cell astrocytoma (SGCA).

SGCAs are low-grade and enhancing solid tumors that are seen in close proximity to the foramen of Monro in the setting of tuberous sclerosis.

Other choices and discussion
A–C, E. Gangliogliomas, PXAs, and DIAs typically present as cystic lesions with enhancing mural nodules. The "cyst with dot" sign can be seen in the vesicular and colloidal vesicular stages of neurocysticercosis.

References

Daghistani R, Miller E, Kulkarni AV, et al. Atypical characteristics and behavior of dysembryoplastic neuroepithelial tumors. *Neuroradiology*. 2013;55(2):217–224.

Dudley RW, Torok MR, Gallegos DR, et al. Pediatric low-grade ganglioglioma: epidemiology, treatments, and outcome analysis on 348 children from the surveillance, epidemiology and end results database. *Neurosurgery*. 2015;76(3):313–319.

Case 32

Please refer to the following images to answer the next three questions:

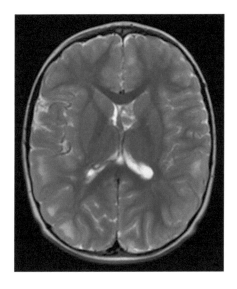 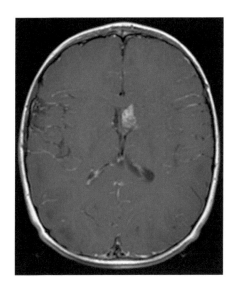

A 6-year-old male with seizure disorder.

32.1 What is the **MOST** likely diagnosis?

A. Central neurocytoma.

B. Intraventricular meningioma.

C. Subependymal giant cell astrocytoma (SEGA).

D. Subependymoma.

E. Metastasis.

32.2 Which of the following statements is **TRUE** regarding this entity?

A. High-grade neoplasm.

B. Short-interval (3 month) imaging follow-up is necessary.

C. Always deemed a surgical candidate.

D. Rarely calcifies.

E. Surgical resection is curative.

32.3 What imaging parameter differentiates subependymal giant cell astrocytomas from subependymal tubers?

A. Size.

B. Enhancement.

C. Calcification.

D. Location.

E. Central necrosis.

Answers and Explanations

32.1 Correct: C. Subependymal giant cell astrocytoma (SEGA).

Multiple subcortical nonenhancing lesions are seen on the T2-weighted image, which should raise the suspicion for tuberous sclerosis in a young child with a history of seizures. These lesions likely represent a combination of subcortical tubers and white matter radial migration lines composed of glia along the path of neuronal cortical migration. In addition, a heterogenous, enhancing lesion measuring greater than 1 cm is seen along the left foramen of Monro. In the setting of tuberous sclerosis, this lesion is pathognomonic for a SEGA.

Other choices and discussion

A, B, D, E. The other answer choices can present as intraventricular tumors but are less likely in the setting of tuberous sclerosis.

32.2 Correct: E. Surgical resection is curative.

SEGAs are WHO grade I noninfiltrative astrocytomas that can be entirely removed with surgical resection.

Other choices and discussion

A. SEGAs are low grade WHO grade 1 tumors.

B. SEGAs are slow-growing lesions and, hence, short-term (3 month) imaging is not a primary recommendation for follow-up.

C. SEGAs are not always surgically resected. Symptomatic lesions, causing seizures or epilepsy or those causing obstructive hydrocephalus, often require surgical intervention. Lesions that demonstrate progressive growth on serial imaging can also be considered for resection.

D. SEGAs commonly contain calcifications, which is similar to the widespread tubers that are seen in various locations in tuberous sclerosis.

32.3 Correct: A. Size.

In the setting of tuberous sclerosis, enhancing subependymal lesions measuring greater than 1 to 1.3 cm are considered SEGAs. Lesions are categorized as subependymal tubers/nodules if they do not meet this size criteria and are monitored with serial imaging. Small subependymal tubers can be located at the foramen of Monro, similar to SEGAs. Both tubers and SEGAs can enhance and calcify.

Other choices and discussion

B, C. Both SEGAs and tubers can enhance and calcify.

D. Small subependymal tubers can be located at the foramen of Monro, similar to SEGAs.

E. Central necrosis is not a common imaging feature of either lesion.

References

Baskin HJ Jr. The pathogenesis and imaging of the tuberous sclerosis complex. *Pediatr Radiol.* 2008;38(9):936–952.

Manoukian SB, Kowal DJ. Comprehensive imaging manifestations of tuberous sclerosis. *AJR Am J Roentgenol.* 2015;204(5):933–943.

Case 33

Please refer to the following images to answer the next three questions:

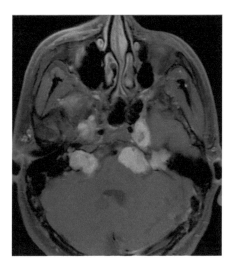 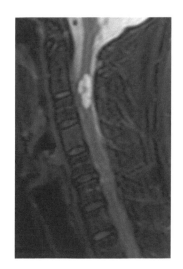

A 31-year-old male presenting with worsening extremity paresthesias.

33.1 What is the **MOST** likely diagnosis on the second image?

A. Schwannoma.

B. Astrocytoma.

C. Ependymoma.

D. Meningioma.

E. Ganglioglioma.

33.2 Which of the following statements regarding neurofibromatosis (NF) type II is **TRUE**?

A. Children with incidental meningioma should undergo testing for NF type II.

B. No imaging follow-up necessary after initial diagnosis. Schwannomas associated with NF type II are WHO grade II tumors.

C. Schwannomas associated with NF type II are WHO grade II tumors.

D. The oculomotor nerve represents the second most common involved cranial nerve.

E. The majority of cases are familial.

33.3 Which of the following imaging features may distinguish a spinal ependymoma from an astrocytoma?

A. Nodular enhancement.

B. Peripheral hemosiderin rim.

C. Tumoral cyst.

D. Syrinx.

E. Peritumoral edema.

Answers and Explanations

33.1   Correct: C. Ependymoma.

The first (postcontrast T1-weighted) image demonstrates large, lobulated, and enhancing extra-axial masses within the internal auditory canals and cerebellopontine angles bilaterally, which are consistent with vestibular schwannomas. Bilateral vestibular schwannomas are pathognomonic for neurofibromatosis (NF) type II. Additional schwannomas are also seen within the Meckel's caves along the trigeminal nerves. NF type II is characterized on imaging by Multiple Inherited Schwannomas, Meningiomas and Ependymomas ("MISs ME lesions"). The second (T2-weighted) image demonstrates a cystic intramedullary tumor. Given the intracranial findings and patient's age, ependymoma is the most likely diagnosis.

Other choices and discussion
B, E. Astrocytomas and gangliogliomas represent intramedullary tumors; however, they are usually seen in the pediatric population and are not as strongly associated with NF type II.
A, D. Although multiple scattered schwannomas and meningiomas can be seen within the spinal canal in NF type II, these are frequently extramedullary in location.

33.2   Correct: A. Children with incidental meningioma should undergo testing for NF type II.

Meningiomas do not usually present in childhood and, hence, should raise the concern for NF type II. These patients should undergo testing, especially if there is a known family history, since meningiomas tend to manifest earlier than other stigmata of NF type II including vestibular schwannomas.

Other choices and discussion
B–E. These options are incorrect. Imaging follow-up option (**B**) is often necessary in order to evaluate for enlarging tumors, compression of vital intracranial structures, worsening vasogenic edema related to meningiomas, and posttreatment status. Schwannomas associated with NF type II (**C**) are histopathologically WHO grade I tumors, similar to incidental schwannomas, but may have a higher proliferative activity. The trigeminal nerves represent the second most common involved cranial nerve instead of oculomotor nerves (**D**). Approximately 50% of cases are familial and autosomal dominant, while 50% are sporadic cases related to new mutations (**E**).

33.3   Correct: B. Peripheral hemosiderin rim.

It is often difficult to distinguish spinal cord ependymomas from astrocytomas due to overlapping imaging features. Cord ependymomas, however, have a propensity to bleed and can present with a hemosiderin "cap sign." This feature may be helpful in distinguishing these tumors from astrocytomas, which rarely hemorrhage.

Other choices and discussion
A, C–E. These answer choices are incorrect. Both ependymomas and astrocytomas can demonstrate nodular enhancement, tumoral cysts, cord syrinx, and peritumoral edema.

References

Goutagny S, Bah AB, Henin D, et al. Long-term follow-up of 287 meningiomas in neurofibromatosis type 2 patients: clinical, radiological, and molecular features. *Neuro Oncol.* 2012;14(8):1090–1096.

Matsuo M, Ohno K, Ohtsuka F. Characterization of early onset neurofibromatosis type 2. *Brain Dev.* 2014;36(2):148–152.

Neff BA, Welling DB. Current concepts in the evaluation and treatment of neurofibromatosis type II. *Otolaryngol Clin North Am.* 2005;38(4):671–684.

Ruggieri M, Iannetti P, Polizzi A, et al. Earliest clinical manifestations and natural history of neurofibromatosis type 2 (NF2) in childhood: a study of 24 patients. *Neuropediatrics.* 2005;36(1):21–34.

Case 34

Please refer to the following images to answer the next three questions:

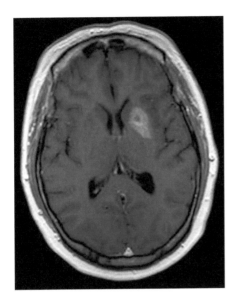
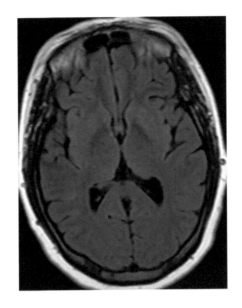

A 32-year-old male with headache.

34.1   What is the **MOST** likely diagnosis?

A. Capillary telangiectasia.

B. Glioma.

C. Metastasis.

D. Developmental venous anomaly.

E. Arteriovenous malformation.

34.2   Which MR sequence is the **MOST** sensitive to confirm the diagnosis?

A. 2D T2* gradient echo (T2* GRE).

B. T1 without contrast.

C. Susceptibility-weighted imaging (SWI).

D. MR angiogram (MRA).

E. T2 single shot fast spin echo (T2 SSFSE).

34.3   What is the **MOST** common location for a capillary telangiectasia?

A. Pons.

B. Cerebellum.

C. Frontal lobe.

D. Medulla.

E. Occipital lobe.

Answers and Explanations

34.1 Correct: A. Capillary telangiectasia.

Postcontrast T1 image demonstrates a "brush-like" enhancing lesion without corresponding T2 fluid-attenuated inversion recovery (FLAIR) signal abnormality centered within the left lentiform nucleus. Capillary telangiectasias, which are clusters of thin-walled capillaries located within the normal brain parenchyma, represent 15 to 20% of low-flow intracranial vascular malformations that do not demonstrate arteriovenous shunting. Larger lesions are drained by a prominent "collector" vein seen on the postcontrast T1 image as an enhancing linear structure along the medial aspect of the lesion. Other low-flow vascular lesions include cavernous malformations and developmental venous anomalies.

Other choices and discussion

B, C. Glioma and metastasis are incorrect because the lesion does not demonstrate mass-like heterogenous enhancement and does not have any associated T2 FLAIR signal abnormality.

D. Although a developmental venous anomaly represents a low-flow vascular malformation, it typically has a large draining cortical vein and a network of smaller veins ("caput medusae" sign) that traverse normal brain parenchyma. Large developmental venous anomalies can cause venous congestion and ischemia within the draining parenchyma and cause signal changes on T2 FLAIR images.

E. An arteriovenous malformation is a high-flow vascular lesion which has a nidus that is typically supplied by hypertrophied arteries and drained by dilated veins findings which are not seen in this case.

34.2 Correct: C. Susceptibility-weighted imaging (SWI).

SWI is a high-resolution, three-dimensional GRE MR sequence which is very sensitive to local disruption of the magnetic field. Sluggish blood flow through the capillary telangiectasia allows conversion of oxyhemoglobin to deoxyhemoglobin which is paramagnetic and distorts the local magnetic field, causing a drop in signal on SWI. Therefore, capillary telangiectasias are seen as hypointense lesions on SWI.

Other choices and discussion

A. Although 2D T2* GRE is also sensitive to local disruption of the magnetic field, three-dimensional SWI has a much greater sensitivity and hence is the correct answer choice.

B and **E.** T1 without contrast and T2 SSFSE are incorrect since capillary telangiectasias generally are not visible on these sequences.

D. MRA can assess for arteriovenous malformations (AVMs) and developmental venous anomalies but capillary telangiectasias are frequently occult on angiographic imaging.

34.3 Correct: A. Pons.

The most common and classic location for a capillary telangiectasia is the pons.

Other choices and discussion

B, D. The cerebellum, medulla, and spinal cord follow the pons in list are less common locations than the pons.

C, E. Up to 30% of lesions can be seen in the supratentorial brain parenchyma.

References

Chaudhry US, De Bruin DE, Policeni BA. Susceptibility-weighted MR imaging: a better technique in the detection of capillary telangiectasia compared with T2* gradient-echo. *AJNR Am J Neuroradiol.* 2014;35(12): 2302–2305.

Gelal F, Karakaş L, Sarsilmaz A, et al. Capillary telangiectasia of the brain: imaging with various magnetic resonance techniques. *JBR-BTR.* 2014;97(4):233–238.

Case 35

Please refer to the following images to answer the next three questions:

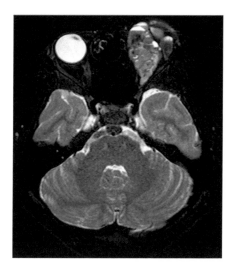 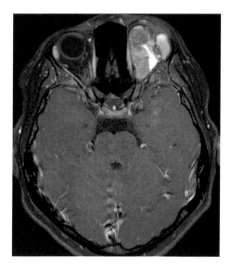

A 9-month-old with left globe proptosis.

35.1 The area of enhancement on the second image represents:

A. Lymphatic tissue.

B. Infection.

C. Vein.

D. Tumor.

E. Fibrosis.

35.2 Which of the imaging findings on CT is highly specific for a venolymphatic malformation?

A. Fluid level.

B. Varix.

C. Soft tissue nodule.

D. Phlebolith.

E. Enhancement.

35.3 Which of the following statements regarding orbital venolymphatic malformations is **TRUE**?

A. Acute intralesional hemorrhage is uncommon.

B. Lesions can increase in size during upper respiratory infections.

C. Majority of the lesions present in young adults.

D. Recurrence after surgical removal is rare.

E. Increase in size with Valsalva.

Answers and Explanations

35.1 Correct: C. Vein.

The first (T2-weighted) image demonstrates a soft-tissue lesion containing multiple fluidfluid levels within the left orbit, which is highly suggestive of a lymphatic malformation. The second (postcontrast T1-weighted) image demonstrates an enhancing tubular structure which is indicative of a venous component to this lesion. Together these findings are diagnostic of a left orbital venolymphatic malformation.

Other choices and discussion

A, B, D, E. The lymphatic components do not enhance (**A**). No inflammatory stranding or abscess is present to suggest infection (**B**). No mass-like lesion is present to suggest tumor (**D**). There are no imaging findings of fibrosis, which typically manifest as T2 hypointense signal (**E**).

35.2 Correct: D. Phlebolith.

The most specific finding of a venous or venolymphatic malformation on CT is a phlebolith. Phleboliths are venous calculi that have a characteristic CT appearance rounded calcifications with lucent centers. Although gonadal vein pheloboliths are a fairly common incidental finding, a soft-tissue lesion containing phleboliths anywhere in the body should raise the concern for a venous or venolymphatic malformation. However, phleboliths are not generally seen in orbital venolymphatic malformations.

Other choices and discussion

A, E. While fluid levels (**A**) and enhancement (**E**) can be seen with venolymphatic malformations; these findings are not as specific as phleboliths.

B. A venous varix is a dilated venous structure that typically increases in size with Valsalva maneuvers. This is not a specific finding of venolymphatic malformations.

C. Venolymphatic malformations typically do not present with soft tissue nodules.

35.3 Correct: B. Lesions can increase in size during upper respiratory tract infections.

Lymphatic components within venolymphatic malformations can reactively increase in size during upper respiratory tract infections.

Other choices and discussion

A. Acute intralesional hemorrhage is not uncommon and can lead to rapid enlargement of the venolymphatic malformation, causing optic nerve compromise, which can subsequently lead to blindness.

C. The majority of the lesions present during childhood and up to 60% of lesions manifest themselves by the mid-teen years.

D. Recurrence after surgical removal is common and seen in up to 50% of cases due to the infiltrative nature of the lesion.

E. Although venolymphatic malformations and orbital varices are related lesions, unlike orbital varices, venolymphatic malformations are hemodynamically isolated and do not increase in size with Valsalva.

References

Chadha V, Awan MA, Gonzalez R, et al. Orbital venous-lymphatic malformation. *Eye* (Lond). 2009;23(12):2265–2266.

Koch BL, Hamilton BE, Hudgins PA, et al. *Diagnostic Imaging: Head and Neck.* 3rd ed. Elsevier; 2017:798–801.

Smoker WR, Lindell GR, Yee NK, et al. Vascular Lesions of the Orbit: More than Meets the Eye. *RadioGraphics.* 2008;28(1):185–204.

Case 36

Please refer to the following images to answer the next three questions:

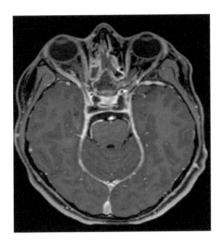

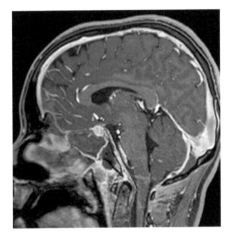

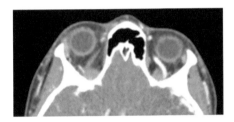

A 14-year-old otherwise healthy female presents with fevers and visual symptoms.

36.1 What is the **MOST** likely diagnosis?

A. Meningitis.

B. Arterial thrombus.

C. Optic neuritis.

D. Cavernous sinus thrombosis.

E. Orbital cellulitis.

36.2 What is the **MOST** likely etiology for the imaging findings?

A. Viral infection.

B. Autoimmune demyelination.

C. Sepsis.

D. Pneumonia.

E. Acute sinusitis.

36.3 Which of the following statements regarding acute invasive fungal sinusitis is **TRUE**?

A. Nonenhancement of sinus mucosa may be seen.

B. Seen in both healthy and immunocompromised individuals.

C. Hyperdense material within the sinuses is a hallmark finding.

D. Medical management is the mainstay of treatment.

E. Associated with low-mortality rate if aggressively treated.

Answers and Explanations

36.1 Correct: D. Cavernous sinus thrombosis.

The axial postcontrast MR image shows lack of contrast enhancement within the cavernous sinuses, which are prominent and exert some degree of mass effect on the cavernous carotid arteries. These findings are concerning for cavernous sinus thrombosis. The sagittal postcontrast image demonstrates opacification of the sphenoid sinus with an abnormal low-T1 signal within the clivus as well as a rim-enhancing fluid collection along its ventral margin. The axial postcontrast CT image demonstrates lack of contrast opacification of the right superior ophthalmic vein (compared to the other side), which is suggestive of thrombosis. Collectively, the imaging findings are concerning for aggressive acute sinusitis, causing central skull base osteomyelitis, abscess, and cavernous sinus thrombosis, with thrombosis extending into the right superior ophthalmic vein.

Other choices and discussion

A–C, E. No specific imaging findings are seen to support the other diagnoses.

36.2 Correct: E. Acute sinusitis.

As discussed in the previous question, there is complete opacification of the sphenoid sinus consistent with acute sinusitis. There is concurrent central skull base osteomyelitis as evidenced by marrow signal abnormality of the clivus and an adjacent abscess.

Other choices and discussion

A. Bacterial infection is the microorganism responsible causing the imaging findings.

B. There are no imaging findings of demyelination. The white matter in the brain is preserved.

C, D. The cause of cavernous sinus thrombosis is usually an infection. While sepsis (**C**) and pneumonia (**D**) are infectious processes, cavernous sinus thrombosis is typically a late complication of an infection of the central face, paranasal sinuses, or teeth. Findings of sphenoid sinusitis with complicating abscess and skull base osteomyelitis are present in this case.

36.3 Correct: A. Nonenhancement of sinus mucosa may be seen.

Nonenhancement of the sinus mucosa can be seen with acute invasive fungal sinusitis. In fact, lack of contrast enhancement has been associated with a poorer prognosis. Areas of nonenhancement have also been shown to correspond with high fungal load with areas of coagulation necrosis.

Other choices and discussion

B. Acute invasive fungal sinusitis is mainly seen in immunocompromised patients such as uncontrolled diabetics, patients afflicted with neutropenia, and AIDS. It tends to be very aggressive and often rapidly infiltrates the orbits and skull base.

C. Hyperdense material within the sinuses usually indicate inspissated secretions or fungal colonization, which can be seen with chronic sinus disease or allergic fungal sinusitis. This is not a hallmark finding of acute invasive fungal sinusitis.

D. Despite ongoing medical management, surgical debridement with removal of necrotic infected tissue is the mainstay of treatment.

E. Despite aggressive medical and surgical management, this condition has high morbidity and mortality rates.

References

Aribandi M, McCoy VA, Bazan C. Imaging features of invasive and noninvasive fungal sinusitis: a review. *Radiographics.* 2007;27(5):1283–1296.

Raz E, Win W, Hagiwara M, et al. Fungal sinusitis. *Neuroimaging Clin N Am.* 2015;25(4):569–576.

Case 37

Please refer to the following images to answer the next three questions:

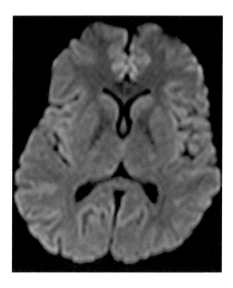 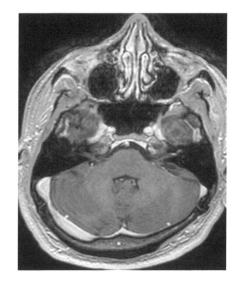

A 40-year-old female presents to the emergent department with abrupt onset of neurological symptoms.

37.1 What is the **MOST** likely presenting clinical symptom in this patient?

A. Right leg weakness.
B. Right facial droop.
C. Left hand numbness.
D. Left facial droop.
E. Left leg weakness.

37.2 What is the imaging follow-up recommendation for this entity?

A. Follow-up contrast MRI in 3 months.
B. No imaging follow-up.
C. Head and neck MRA (MR angiogram).
D. Head MRV (MR venogram).
E. Temporal bone CT.

37.3 Enhancement of which of the following segment of the facial nerve is always considered abnormal?

A. Intraparotid segment.
B. Anterior genu.
C. Tympanic segment.
D. Mastoid segment.
E. Posterior genu.

Answers and Explanations

37.1 Correct: D. Left facial droop.

Postcontrast T1 image demonstrates focal thickening and enhancement of the distal internal auditory canal segment of the left facial nerve ("fundal tuft" sign), which is a classic imaging finding of Bell's palsy. Enhancement of the labyrinthine segment and geniculate ganglion is also observed. The patient would present with unilateral facial droop related to rapid onset of facial nerve paralysis (**D**). Enhancement and thickening of the geniculate ganglion with extension to the meatal, labyrinthine, and anterior tympanic segments is typically seen in Bell's palsy, although the entire nerve can be involved. Findings are related to reactivation of latent herpes simplex infection within the geniculate ganglion. Nodular enhancement should raise the concern for an underlying mass lesion such as a schwannoma.

Other choices and discussion

B. No abnormal enhancement is seen along the visualized right facial nerve and hence this answer choice is incorrect.

A, C, E. The other answer choices are incorrect since no acute infarct or other acute brain parenchymal abnormality is seen on the diffusion-weighted imaging (DWI).

37.2 Correct: B. No imaging follow-up.

The majority (90%) of patients recover within 2 months of symptom onset. Treatment includes steroid therapy and symptomatic management. Antivirals are no longer recommended. No imaging follow-up is necessary. In fact, no imaging is recommended at initial presentation, if the patient presents with typical symptoms of Bell's palsy. However, in clinical practice, imaging is often performed to exclude an acute infarct.

Other choices and discussion

A. Follow-up MRI is not needed in classic Bell's palsy.

C–E. Further imaging with MRA (**C**), MRV (**D**), or temporal bone CT (**E**) are not necessary and would be of limited utility in classic Bell's palsy.

37.3 Correct: A. Intraparotid segment.

Enhancement of the intraparotid segment is always considered abnormal and could be related to a facial nerve schwannoma, but one should always scrutinize the parotid gland for a primary tumor associated with perineural spread of tumor along the facial nerve.

Other choices and discussion

B–E. The geniculate ganglion (anterior genu) (**B**), posterior genu (junction between the tympanic and mastoid segments) (**E**), tympanic (**C**), and mastoid (**D**) portions of the facial nerve can normally demonstrate mild, linear enhancement related to the facial arteriovenous plexus. However, prominent asymmetric enhancement, especially with nerve thickening, of the normally enhancing segments is abnormal. The cisternal, meatal, and intraparotid portions should not normally enhance.

References

Hohman MH, Hadlock TA. Etiology, diagnosis, and management of facial palsy: 2000 patients at a facial nerve center. *The Laryngoscope*. 2014;124:E283–E293.

Zandian A, Osiro S, Hudson R, et al. The neurologist's dilemma: a comprehensive clinical review of Bell's palsy, with emphasis on current management trends. *Med Sci Monit*. 2014;20:83–90.

Case 38

Please refer to the following images to answer the next three questions:

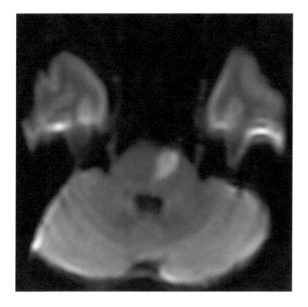

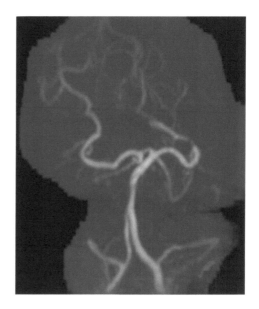

A 63-year-old male with extremity weakness.

38.1 What is the **MOST** likely cause of this patient's symptoms?

A. Moyamoya.

B. Demyelination.

C. Dissection.

D. Vasculitis.

E. Atherosclerosis.

38.2 Which of the following statements regarding this lesion is **TRUE**?

A. It can lead to hypertrophy of the olivary nucleus.

B. It is related to rapid correction of hyponatremia.

C. It can enhance up to four months from the time of the initial insult.

D. Symptoms can include contralateral cranial nerve palsy and ipsilateral hemiplegia.

E. It is also called Wallenberg syndrome.

38.3 Which of the following statements regarding vessel wall imaging is **TRUE**?

A. Vessel wall imaging can be used to differentiate between radiation-induced arteriopathy and inflammatory vasculitis.

B. Vessel wall imaging can reliably detect peripheral branch vessel vasculitis.

C. The hallmark imaging finding in reverse cerebral vasoconstriction syndrome (RCVS) is avid vessel wall enhancement.

D. Proton-density-weighted sequences (PDWS) can be obtained instead of T1 due to the higher signal-to-noise ratio (SNR).

E. Two-dimensional acquisition can be used to identify any inflammatory vascular disease, while three-dimensional imaging can target a known lesion for better characterization given the higher in-plane spatial resolution.

Answers and Explanations

38.1 Correct: E. Atherosclerosis.

The diffusion-weighted imaging (DWI) demonstrates an acute infarct within the territory of a pontine perforator branch vessel, which is likely related to underlying small vessel atherosclerosis and occlusion. The three-dimensional reformatted time-of-flight MR angiographic image of the posterior circulation demonstrates only mild narrowing of the midbasilar artery, and focal moderate-to-severe narrowing of the P2P3 junction of the left posterior cerebral artery. There is mild atherosclerotic irregularity of some of the other branch vessels.

Other choices and discussion
C. No significant irregularity or high-grade stenosis of the basilar artery is present to raise concerns about an underlying dissection (**C**).
A, B, D. No additional history or imaging is provided to support the diagnosis of other answer choices. Central pontine myelinolysis represents acute osmotic demyelination (**B**) of the brainstem white matter tracts related to rapid correction of hyponatremia. This lesion can restrict but, unlike a pontine perforator infarct, it presents as a symmetric central brainstem T2 hyperintense lesion with sparing of the periphery. Moyamoya vasculopathy (**A**) generally spares the posterior circulation, especially the basilar artery. Although vascular irregularity and multifocal narrowing can be imaging manifestations of vasculitis (**D**), without the supporting clinical information and additional images, the most common cause of such imaging findings in an older patient is intracranial atherosclerosis.

38.2 Correct: A. It can lead to hypertrophy of the olivary nucleus.

An infarct within the brainstem that disrupts the central tegmental tract (which is part of the dentato-rubro-olivary connection and also known as the triangle of Guillain and Mollaret) can lead to hypertrophy of the inferior olivary nucleus.

Other choices and discussion
B–E. Answer choice (**B**) is incorrect since this lesion represents an acute infarct rather than osmotic demyelination. Infarcts within the subacute phase have been reported to enhance up to 2 to 3 months from the time of the primary insult and not 4 months (**C**), when infarcts are generally considered to be in the chronic stage. Brainstem infarcts can lead to *unilateral* cranial nerve palsies and *contralateral* hemiparesis. Hence, answer choice (**D**) is incorrect. In Wallenberg syndrome (**E**), infarcts involve the lateral medulla, and not pons, and are related to occlusion of the intracranial vertebral artery or posterior inferior cerebellar artery.

38.3 Correct: D. Proton-density-weighted sequences (PDWS) can be obtained instead of T1 due to the higher signal-to-noise ratio (SNR).

Vessel wall MRA represents high-resolution, postcontrast imaging of the intracranial arteries with utilization of various MR techniques to suppress the signal from luminal blood and cerebrospinal fluid (CSF) in order to allow characterization of the arterial walls and to assess for underlying inflammation. PDWS can be utilized for this purpose since they have a higher SNR than T1-weighted images; however, vessel wall enhancement can be less conspicuous on PDFS imaging which is a major drawback of this technique.

Other choices and discussion
A–C, E. Answer choice (**A**) is incorrect since both inflammatory vasculitis and radiation-induced arteriopathy can appear identical on vessel wall imaging obtained at a single time point, with both entities potentially showing avid circumferential enhancement of the vessel walls. Vessel wall enhancement can persist in radiation-induced arteriopathy for many years, whereas it tends to resolve in inflammatory vasculitis upon clinical resolution of the inciting cause. The spatial resolution and SNR on 3 Tesla MRI, the highest magnetic strength used in clinical practice currently, is not high enough to reliably diagnose small-vessel vasculitis involving peripheral intracranial branch vessels (**B**). The key distinguishing feature of RCVs from vasculitis on vessel wall imaging is lack of avid arterial wall enhancement, though both conditions present with vessel wall thickening. Hence, answer choice (**C**) is incorrect. Three-dimensional vessel wall imaging is a faster technique compared to two-dimensional imaging since it utilizes an isotropic voxel and can be reformatted in any plane. However, the in-plane spatial resolution of two-dimensional imaging is higher. Therefore, three-dimensional imaging can be obtained initially to detect any abnormal vascular disease and two-dimensional sequences can target any detected vascular disease for better characterization (**E**).

References

Gao T, Yu W, Liu C. Mechanisms of ischemic stroke in patients with intracranial atherosclerosis: A high-resolution magnetic resonance imaging study. Exp Ther Med. 2014;7(5):1415–1419.

Lindenholz A, Van Der Kolk AG, Zwanenburg JJ, et al. The Use and Pitfalls of Intracranial Vessel Wall Imaging: How We Do It. Radiology. 2017;286(1):12–28.

Mandell DM, Mossa-Basha M, Qiao Y, et al. Intracranial Vessel Wall MRI: Principles and Expert Consensus Recommendations of the American Society of Neuroradiology. *AJNR Am J Neuroradiol.* 2017;38(2):218–229.

Case 39

Please refer to the following images to answer the next three questions:

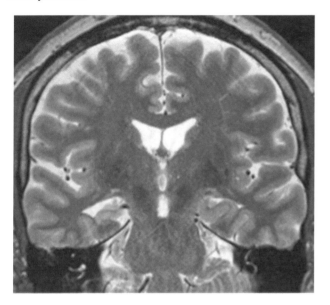

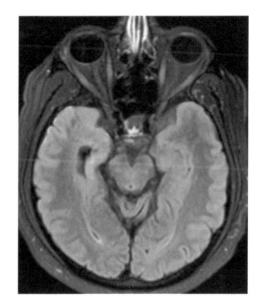

A 47-year-old male with history of temporal lobe epilepsy.

39.1 Which of the following sequences is the **MOST** sensitive for evaluation of hippocampal internal architecture?

A. T1.
B. Gradient echo (GRE).
C. Spin echo T2.
D. Two-dimensional fluid-attenuated inversion recovery (FLAIR).
E. Three-dimensional (FLAIR).

39.2 With regard to structural involvement in mesial temporal sclerosis, what is the **CORRECT** order of frequency (highest to lowest)?

A. Mamillary body > fornix > amygdala > hippocampus.
B. Hippocampus > fornix > mamillary body > amygdala.
C. Amygdala > fornix > hippocampus > mamillary body.
D. Fornix > hippocampus > amygdala > mamillary body.
E. Hippocampus > amygdala > fornix > mamillary body.

39.3 Which of the following statements is **TRUE** regarding mesial temporal sclerosis?

A. 50% of cases are bilateral.
B. fMRI is replacing Wada testing for localization of language function.
C. Normal or elevated NAA seen on spectroscopy.
D. Surgical resection is the mainstay of treatment.
E. CA2 and CA3 are the most susceptible to damage.

Answers and Explanations

39.1   Correct: C. Spin echo T2.

The images demonstrate T2/FLAIR hyperintensity within the right hippocampal head and body with volume loss and loss of the normal internal architecture–findings which are compatible with mesial temporal sclerosis. Coronal spin echo T2-weighted images are the most sensitive for evaluation of the hippocampal internal architecture, while coronal FLAIR images are most sensitive for assessing the underlying signal abnormality. Both two-dimensional and three-dimensional FLAIR sequences can be used to assess for signal changes, although subtle signal changes may be better seen with a high-resolution three-dimensional sequence.

Other choices and discussion
A, B, D, E. Other answer choices are incorrect. T1-weighted images are less revealing than T2 or FLAIR images. GRE sequences can be obtained to assess for an underlying hemorrhagic lesion, such as a cavernous malformation; however, the hippocampal structure is not well-evaluated on GRE.

39.2   Correct: E. Hippocampus > amygdala > fornix > mamillary body.

The hippocampus is the most commonly involved structure in mesial temporal sclerosis. The amygdala is the second most commonly involved structure. Forniceal and mamillary body involvement is less common but can be seen with advanced mesial temporal sclerosis.

Other choices and discussion
The order of structures in answer choices (**A–D**) are incorrect. The hippocampus is most commonly involved in mesial temporal sclerosis making (**A**), (**C**), and (**D**) incorrect. The amygdala is the second most commonly involved structure, making (**B**) incorrect.

39.3   Correct: B. fMRI is replacing Wada testing for localization of language function.

Improved fMRI techniques allow for reliable localization of the language centers and is increasingly replacing Wada testing as the noninvasive test of choice.

Other choices and discussion
A, C–E. The other answer choices are incorrect. Only 10 to 20% of cases are bilateral. Decreased NAA is seen within the affected temporal lobe on spectroscopy. Medical management is the mainstay of treatment. CA1 and CA4 are the most commonly affected regions of the hippocampal formation.

References

Azab M, Carone M, Ying S, et al. Mesial Temporal Sclerosis: Accuracy of NeuroQuant versus Neuroradiologist. *AJNR Am J Neuroradiol.* 2015;36(8):1400–1406.

Blumcke I, Coras R, Miyata H, et al. Defining clinic-neuropathological subtypes of mesial temporal lobe epilepsy with hippocampal sclerosis. *Brain Pathol.* 2012;22(3):402–411.

Malmgren K, Thom M. Hippocampal sclerosis-origins and imaging. *Epilepsia.* 2012;53 Suppl 4:19–33.

Case 40

Please refer to the following images to answer the next three questions:

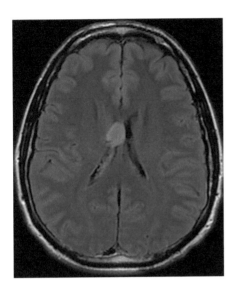
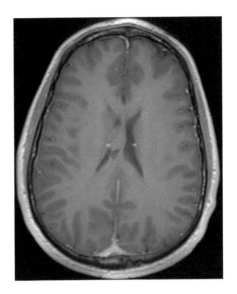

A 37-year-old male presents with headache and neck pain 2 days after motor vehicle collision.

40.1 The lesion depicted can physiologically behave similar to which of the following entities?

A. Glioblastoma.

B. Medulloblastoma.

C. Pituitary microadenoma.

D. Cavernous malformation.

E. Colloid cyst.

40.2 Which of the following statements regarding subependymomas is **TRUE**?

A. Majority of the lesions demonstrate avid enhancement.

B. Present as parenchymal masses within the supratentorial brain.

C. Typically seen in the setting of tuberous sclerosis.

D. Asymptomatic lesions can be followed-up with serial imaging.

E. Commonly affect young males.

40.3 Which of the following imaging features would be atypical for a central neurocytoma?

A. No enhancement.

B. Bubbly appearance.

C. Calcification.

D. Hydrocephalus.

E. Internal flow voids.

Answers and Explanations

40.1   Correct: E. Colloid cyst.

The first image demonstrates a solid fluid-attenuated inversion recovery (FLAIR) hyperintense ovoid mass within the body of the right lateral ventricle, abutting the septum pellucidum.

Other choices and discussion

E. Given the close proximity to the foramen on Monro, this lesion can cause obstructive hydrocephalus, which can be seen with a third ventricular colloid cyst (**E**).

A–D. The other lesions usually do not present in this location.

40.2   Correct: D. Asymptomatic lesions can be followed-up with serial imaging.

Asymptomatic subependymomas can be followed-up with serial imaging, especially if the risks of surgical resection outweigh the benefits.

Other choices and discussion

A–C, E. The other answer choices are incorrect. The majority of subependymomas demonstrate mild-to-no significant enhancement and rarely present as avidly enhancing tumors. The most common location for a subependymoma is the 4th ventricle, followed by the lateral ventricles. Supratentorial *ependymomas* generally present as large parenchymal masses. Subependymal giant cell astrocytoma (SEGA), a histologically distinct tumor, is typically seen in patients with tuberous sclerosis. The prototypical patient presenting with a symptomatic or incidental subependymoma is an elderly male.

40.3   Correct: A. No enhancement.

The majority of central neurocytomas demonstrate moderate-to-marked enhancement. Lack of enhancement is unusual and raises the probability that the lesion is instead a subependymoma.

Other choices and discussion

B. A "bubbly" heterogenous mass within the body of the lateral ventricle is a good diagnostic clue for a central neurocytoma, which is often related to underlying cystic areas.

C. Internal calcifications are also fairly common, occurring in up to 70% of cases.

D, E. Central neurocytomas can vary from being avascular to hypervascular (**E**)—internal flow voids may be seen in hypervascular central neurocytomas and can be confirmed on conventional angiography. Since central neurocytomas are commonly adherent to the septum pellucidum and in close proximity to the foramen of Monro, they can present clinically with obstructive hydrocephalus (**D**).

References

Bi Z, Ren X, Zhang J, et al. Clinical, radiological, and pathological features in 43 cases of intracranial subependymoma. *J Neurosurg.* 2015;122(1)49–60.

Donoho D, Zada G. Imaging of central neurocytomas. *Neurosurg Clin N Am.* 2015;26(1):11–19.

Case 41

Please refer to the following images to answer the next three questions:

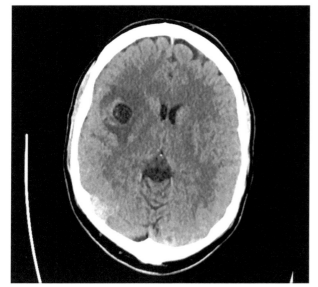

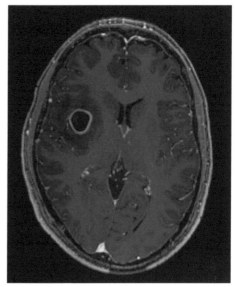

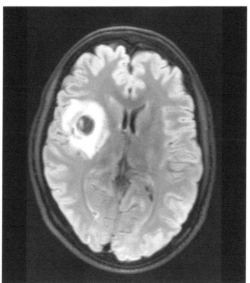

A 20-year-old female presents with new onset of seizures.

41.1 What is the **MOST** likely diagnosis?

A. Enlarged perivascular space.

B. Multiple sclerosis.

C. Sarcoidosis.

D. Neurocysticercosis.

E. DNET (dysembryoplastic neuroepithelial tumor).

41.2 Which pathologic stage is demonstrated here?

A. Vesicular stage.

B. Active nodular stage.

C. Nodular calcified stage.

D. Granular nodular stage.

E. Colloidal vesicular stage.

41.3 What is the **MOST** common central nervous system site for this diagnosis?

A. Convexity subarachnoid space.

B. Ventricles.

C. Parenchyma.

D. Basal cisterns.

E. Orbit.

Answers and Explanations

41.1   Correct: D. Neurocysticercosis.

On the axial noncontrast CT image, a round hypodense lesion with surrounding vasogenic edema is demonstrated; on close inspection, an internal punctate hyperdensity is present which represents a scolex. This appearance of a cyst with a scolex is pathognomonic for neurocysticercosis. Seizures secondary to inflammation from degenerating larvae are the most common presenting symptoms.

Other choices and discussion

A. An enlarged perivascular space is unlikely given the extensive surrounding vasogenic edema.
B. Peripherally enhancing lesions which are seen in active demyelinating plaques of multiple sclerosis demonstrate an incomplete rim of enhancement, not complete as seen here.
C. Sarcoidosis most commonly presents with leptomeningeal or dural enhancement, and a cystic appearance in the parenchyma is atypical.
E. A "bubbly" T2 hyperintense and cortically based mass in a patient with more long-standing seizures is typical of DNET, which is not seen or reported here.

41.2   Correct: E. Colloidal vesicular stage.

Neurocysticercosis can be classified into four stages, with each stage possessing a characteristic imaging appearance. In the colloidal vesicular stage (shown here), the larva and associated scolex degenerate, which trigger an inflammatory response with peripheral enhancement of the cyst wall and a large amount of vasogenic edema.

Other choices and discussion

A. In the vesicular stage, the infection is quiescent, and there is a smooth, thin-walled cyst with no wall enhancement and surrounding edema. In the colloidal vesicular stage, the larva and associated scolex are degenerating which trigger an inflammatory response, and there is peripheral enhancement of the cyst walls and a large amount of vasogenic edema.
B. There is no active nodular stage in neurocysticercosis.
D. In the granular nodular stage, healing is occurring, so there is only minimal enhancement remaining and edema has considerably decreased.
C. In the nodular calcified stage, the infection is no longer active and the residual shrunken nodules will calcify.

41.3   Correct: A. Convexity subarachnoid spaces.

Convexity subarachnoid spaces are the most common location for neurocysticercosis.

Other choices and discussion

D. The next most common location is the basal cisterns, where one can see multilobulated, grape-like lesions in the racemose form of neurocysticercosis.
B, C. The parenchyma **(C)** is the third-most common location, followed by the ventricles **(B)**. Intraventricular cysts are subtle on CT, and fluid-attenuated inversion recovery (FLAIR) and heavily T2-weighted sequences on MRI are helpful in detection.
E. The orbit is rarely involved.

References

Kimura-Hayama ET, Higuera JA, Corona-Cedillo R, et al. Neurocysticercosis: radiologic-pathologic correlation. *Radiographics*. 2010;30(6):1705–1719.

Lucato LT, Guedes MS, Sato JR, et al. The role of conventional MR imaging sequences in the evaluation of neurocysticercosis: impact on characterization of the scolex and lesion burden. *AJNR Am J Neuroradiol*. 2007;28(8):1501-1504.

Osborn AG. Parasitic Infections. In: Osborn AG, Hedlund GL, editors. Osborn's Brain: Imaging, Pathology, and Anatomy. 2nd ed. Philadelphia: Elsevier; 2018: 390–399.

Case 42

Please refer to the following images to answer the next three questions:

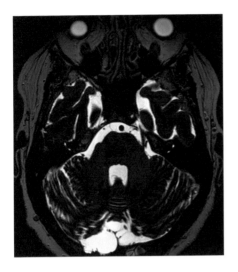
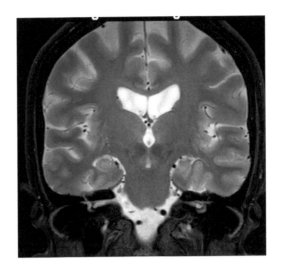

A 60-year-old male with episodic lancinating facial pain.

42.1 What is the **MOST** likely diagnosis?

A. Perineural spread.

B. Trigeminal neuralgia.

C. Aneurysm in cerebellopontine angle.

D. Pontine developmental venous anomaly.

E. Facial nerve schwannoma.

42.2 What is the **MOST** common culprit vessel?

A. Petrosal vein.

B. Trigeminal artery.

C. Basilar artery.

D. Anterior inferior cerebellar artery.

E. Superior cerebellar artery.

42.3 Which of the following can be seen after stereotactic radiosurgery in the treatment of neurovascular compression?

A. Restoration of the bulk of the trigeminal nerve.

B. Focal contrast enhancement of the trigeminal nerve.

C. Transection of the cisternal segment.

D. Worsening of nerve displacement by the offending vessel.

E. Occlusion or high-grade stenosis of the offending vessel.

Answers and Explanations

42.1 Correct: B. Trigeminal neuralgia.

Patients with trigeminal neuralgia report episodic intense stabbing pain in the distribution of the trigeminal nerve. Often the episode is triggered by tactile stimulation of the face by daily activities such as shaving or eating. As seen in this case, neurovascular compression occurring at the root entry zone or preganglionic segment of the trigeminal nerve is the most common etiology for trigeminal neuralgia. Longstanding compression results in atrophy of the cisternal trigeminal nerve, which can sometimes be appreciated on cross-sectional, high-resolution imaging of the nerve.

Other choices and discussion

C–E. Posterior fossa developmental venous anomalies (**D**) and mass lesions such as facial nerve schwannoma (**E**) or aneurysm in the cerebellopontine angle (**C**) can be responsible for facial pain and must be excluded; however, these are not present in this case.
A. Perineural spread is unlikely in the absence of a known primary malignancy, and either abnormal enlargement or enhancement of the cranial nerve would be expected.

42.2 Correct: E. Superior cerebellar artery.

The superior cerebellar artery from above is the most common culprit vessel in neurovascular compression of the trigeminal nerve, occurring in 88% of cases.

Other choices and discussion

A–D. The next most common offending vessel is the anterior inferior cerebellar artery (**D**) from below, occurring in less than 25% of cases. Even more uncommon are the basilar (**C**), vertebral, and persistent trigeminal arteries (**B**) and petrosal vein (**A**).

42.3 Correct: B. Focal contrast enhancement of the trigeminal nerve.

The treated nerve may demonstrate focal contrast enhancement after stereotactic radiosurgery.

Other choices and discussion

A. Atrophy of the treated nerve, rather than increased bulk (**A**), occurs in 96% of patients who undergo stereotactic radiosurgery.
C–E. Nerve transection (**C**), worsening of nerve displacement (**D**), and steno-occlusion (**E**) of the offending vessel are not commonly observed in this setting.

References

Haller S, Etienne L, Kövari E, et al. Imaging of Neurovascular Compression Syndromes: Trigeminal Neuralgia, Hemifacial Spasm, Vestibular Paroxysmia, and Glossopharyngeal Neuralgia. *AJNR Am J Neuroradiol*. 2016;37(8):1384–1392.

Miller J, Acar F, Hamilton B, et al. Preoperative visualization of neurovascular anatomy in trigeminal neuralgia. *J Neurosurg*. 2008;108:477–482.

Case 43

Please refer to the following images to answer the next three questions:

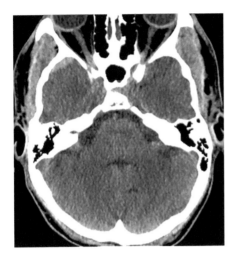 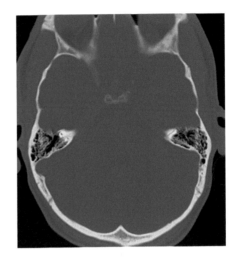

A 24-year-old male presents after being assaulted at a bar.

43.1 What is the **MOST** likely diagnosis?

A. Subdural hematoma.
B. Subarachnoid hemorrhage.
C. Arterial epidural hematoma.
D. Benign anterior temporal epidural hematoma.
E. Hemorrhagic contusion.

43.2 What is the natural history of this entity?

A. Excellent prognosis after surgical evacuation.
B. Rapid expansion and clinical deterioration.
C. Stable size and benign clinical course.
D. Gradual increase in size.
E. Initial stability but with delayed increase in size.

43.3 Which structure is disrupted in this entity?

A. Superior sagittal sinus.
B. Sphenoparietal sinus.
C. Middle meningeal artery.
D. Middle meningeal vein.
E. Basilar venous plexus.

Answers and Explanations

43.1   Correct: D. Benign anterior temporal epidural hematoma.

On the axial CT image with brain window, there is a hyperdense, biconvex, extra-axial hematoma on the right, at the anterior margin of the middle cranial fossa, which is bounded laterally by the sphenotemporal suture. This is a classic imaging appearance for a benign anterior temporal epidural hematoma. On the axial CT image with bone window, there is a minimally displaced fracture of the greater wing of the sphenoid bone. Most anterior temporal epidural hematomas are associated with a fracture of the greater wing of the sphenoid or the zygomaticomaxillary complex.

Other choices and discussion
A. In contrast, a subdural hematoma would be expected to appear crescentic rather than biconvex in shape.
B. Although posttraumatic subarachnoid hemorrhage can be focal, the typical findings of hyperdensity in the Sylvian fissure, cerebral convexity sulci, and interpeduncular cistern are not demonstrated here.
C. The more common arterial epidural hematoma is also biconvex in morphology; however, it typically occurs along the temporoparietal convexity adjacent to the middle meningeal artery groove.
E. A hemorrhagic contusion is intra-axial and not extra-axial in location.

43.2   Correct: C. Stable size and benign clinical course.

The anterior temporal epidural hematoma is usually asymptomatic and remains stable in size over time.

Other choices and discussion
A, B, D, E. Anterior temporal lobe epidural hematomas typically do not increase in size over time (**D**). Surgical evacuation (**A**) is not usually needed, and the patient can be followed clinically. Follow-up CT head imaging can performed in 24 to 36 hours to ensure stability. As this hematoma is located anterior, and not lateral to the temporal lobe, no cerebral herniation, midline shift, or effacement of basilar cisterns occurs. Arterial epidural hematomas are associated with rapid expansion and clinical deterioration (**B**) or initial stability with delayed increase in size (**E**).

43.3   Correct: B. Sphenoparietal sinus.

The sphenoparietal sinus, which is anteriorly located within the middle cranial fossa, is thought to be disrupted, resulting in venous bleeding which forms the anterior temporal epidural hematoma.

Other choices and discussion
A. The superior sagittal sinus is disrupted in a vertex epidural hematoma.
C. The middle meningeal artery is typically injured in an arterial epidural hematoma.
D. While injury of the middle meningeal vein can result in a venous epidural hematoma, injury of the sphenoparietal sinus causes a venous epidural hematoma in the specific location seen in this case.
E. The basilar venous plexus is injured in a clival epidural hematoma.

References

Gean AD, Fischbein NJ, Purcell DD, et al. Benign Anterior Temporal Epidural Hematoma: Indolent Lesion with a Characteristic CT Imaging Appearance after Blunt Head Trauma. *Radiology*. 2010;257(1):212–218.

Sullivan TP, Jarvik JG, Cohen WA. Follow-up of conservatively managed epidural hematomas: implications for timing of repeat CT. *AJNR Am J Neuroradiol*. 1999;20(1):107–113.

Case 44

Please refer to the following images to answer the next three questions:

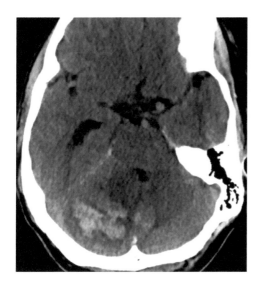 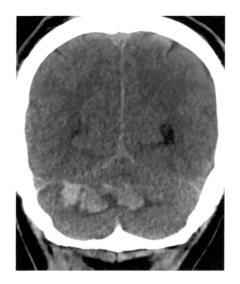

A 60-year-old male who underwent spine hardware removal one day prior now presents with altered mental status.

44.1 What is the **MOST** likely diagnosis?

A. Remote cerebellar hemorrhage.

B. Hemorrhagic metastasis.

C. Hypertensive hemorrhage.

D. Cerebral amyloid angiopathy.

E. LhermitteDuclos disease.

44.2 What is the imaging sign associated with this entity?

A. Hot cross buns sign.

B. Zebra sign.

C. Empty delta sign.

D. White cerebellum sign.

E. Tigroid pattern.

44.3 Which of the following is **TRUE** regarding remote cerebellar hemorrhage (RCH)?

A. RCH occurs more commonly after spinal surgery than supratentorial craniotomy.

B. RCH occurs only ipsilateral to the side of surgery.

C. Pathophysiology is likely attributable to intracranial hypotension secondary to cerebrospinal fluid (CSF) leak.

D. RCH typically occurs within 7 to 10 days after surgery.

E. External ventricular drain placement is a predisposing condition.

Answers and Explanations

44.1   Correct: A. Remote cerebellar hemorrhage.

On the axial and CT images, there is acute hemorrhage in the right greater than left cerebellar hemispheres and vermis; given the clinical history, the image findings are compatible with remote cerebellar hemorrhage occurring as a complication of spinal surgery. The images also demonstrate associated mass effect in the posterior fossa, resulting in obstructive hydrocephalus.

Other choices and discussion

B. In the absence of a history of primary malignancy, hemorrhagic metastasis is a less likely possibility.
C. In the absence of a history of hypertension, hypertensive hemorrhage is less likely.
D. Cerebral amyloid angiopathy is uncommon in the cerebellum.
E. Although LhermitteDuclos disease occurs in the cerebellum, thickening of the cerebellar folia rather than hyperdense hemorrhage in a striated pattern is typically seen.

44.2   Correct: B. Zebra sign.

The zebra sign of remote cerebellar hemorrhage seen in this case reflects hyperdense, acute hemorrhage layering within the cerebellar folia, which creates a striped appearance.

Other choices and discussion

A. The hot cross buns sign refers to cruciform T2 hyperintensity in the pons, reflecting multisystem atrophy.
C. The empty delta sign refers to nonenhancing thrombus in the dural venous sinus on cross-sectional CT images.
D. The white cerebellum sign indicates hypoxemic ischemic brain injury with hypodense appearance of the cerebral hemispheres in comparison to the relatively hyperdense cerebellum.
E. The tigroid pattern is seen in metachromatic leukodystrophy, with dark stripes emanating from the ventricular margins on a background of hyperintense periventricular white matter.

44.3   Correct: C. Pathophysiology is likely attributable to intracranial hypotension secondary to cerebrospinal fluid (CSF) leak.

The pathophysiology of remote cerebellar hemorrhage is uncertain but theorized to be related to intracranial hypotension and brain sagging, occurring as a result of a CSF leak with subsequent occlusion or tearing of bridging veins.

Other choices and discussion

A. RCH occurs more commonly after supratentorial craniotomy than after spinal surgery.
B. RCH occurs contralateral to surgery in 29% of cases.
D. RCH usually occurs within hours to 1 day after spinal surgery as seen in this case.
E. Lumbar drain placement, not external ventricular drain placement, is a predisposing factor.

References

Chavhan GB, Shroff MM. Twenty classic signs in neuroradiology: A pictorial essay *Indian J Radiol Imaging*. 2009;19(2):135–145.

Nam TK, Park SW, Min BK, et al. Remote cerebellar hemorrhage after lumbar spinal surgery. *J Korean Neurosurg Soc*. 2009;46(5):501–504.

Case 45

Please refer to the following images to answer the next three questions:

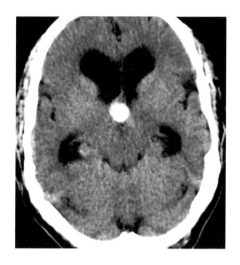

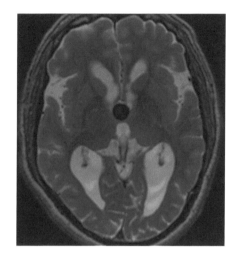

A 60-year-old male presents with intermittent headache.

45.1 What is the **MOST** likely diagnosis?

A. Pituitary apoplexy.

B. Pineal tumor.

C. Colloid cyst.

D. Aneurysm.

E. Choroid plexus papilloma.

45.2 What complication of this entity is demonstrated?

A. Herniation.

B. Obstructive hydrocephalus.

C. Cyst rupture.

D. Hemorrhage.

E. Ventriculitis.

45.3 What is the preferred treatment for this entity?

A. Complete resection.

B. Stereotactic aspiration.

C. Observation.

D. Complete resection if hydrocephalus present, observation otherwise.

E. Ventricular shunt.

Answers and Explanations

45.1 Correct: C. Colloid cyst.

On the axial CT image, there is a round hyperdense lesion, which is located midline at the anterosuperior aspect of the third ventricle, causing obstructive hydrocephalus. On axial T2-weighted MRI, this lesion appears homogeneously hypointense, which is also typical of colloid cysts, although the imaging characteristics can be variable based on the amount of cholesterol and protein contents within the cyst. Nonetheless, the appearance is characteristic of a colloid cyst, and the clinical history of intermittent and positional headaches is the most common presenting symptom of this entity.

Other choices and discussion
A, E, D. Pituitary apoplexy (**A**) and choroid plexus papilloma (**E**) are unlikely in the third ventricle. No phase artifact is seen to suggest aneurysm (**D**).
B. The lesion demonstrated is too far anterior to arise from the pineal gland.

45.2 Correct: B. Obstructive hydrocephalus.

There is moderate diffuse ventriculomegaly with periventricular hyperintensity on T2-weighted imaging consistent with obstructive hydrocephalus that has occurred secondary to the colloid cyst.

Other choices and discussion
A, C–E. There is no evidence of herniation (**A**) or ventriculitis (**E**) on the provided images. No fluidfluid level is present to suggest cyst rupture (**C**) or hemorrhage (**D**).

45.3 Correct: A. Complete resection.

Because colloid cysts can lead to obstructive hydrocephalus, herniation, and even sudden death, complete surgical resection is the most common treatment of choice, and endoscopic approaches are now commonplace.

Other choices and discussion
C. Observation is uncommonly chosen due to the possibility of acute obstruction and death.
D. Surgical resection is the treatment of choice, regardless of whether hydrocephalus is already present.
B, E. Less commonly undertaken treatments are stereotactic aspiration and ventricular shunting.

References

Armao D, Castillo M, Chen H, et al. Colloid Cyst of the Third Ventricle: Imaging-pathologic Correlation. *AJNR Am J Neuroradiol.* 2000;21(8):1470–1477.

Maeder PP, Holtås SL, Basibüyük LN, et al. Colloid cysts of the third ventricle: correlation of MR and CT findings with histology and chemical analysis. *AJNR Am J Neuroradiol.* 1990;11(3):575–581.

Case 46

Please refer to the following images to answer the next three questions:

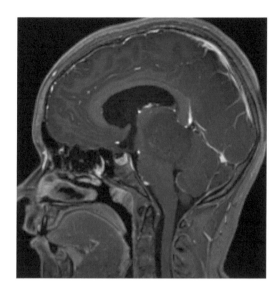

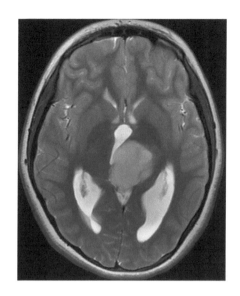

A 10-year-old female presents with Parinaud syndrome and headaches.

46.1 What is the **MOST** characteristic component of Parinaud syndrome?

A. Bitemporal hemianopsia.

B. Upgaze palsy.

C. Seizures.

D. Ptosis.

E. Internuclear ophthalmoplegia.

46.2 What is the **MOST** likely diagnosis?

A. Medulloblastoma.

B. Glioblastoma.

C. Diffuse midline glioma, H3 K27M-mutant.

D. Cavernous malformation.

E. Artery of Percheron infarct.

46.3 Which of the following is **TRUE** of this diagnosis?

A. Nonenhancement is required for the diagnosis.

B. Imaging of the neuraxis is indicated.

C. The H3 K27M mutation confers a better prognosis than the wildtype.

D. H3 K27M-mutant gliomas only occur in children.

E. Indolent lesion with stable appearance over years.

Answers and Explanations

46.1 Correct: B. Upgaze palsy.

Parinaud syndrome (dorsal midbrain syndrome) results from a posterior commissure mass, causing compression of the tectal plate at the level of the superior colliculus, and presents with upgaze palsy (diplopia), pupillary light-near dissociation (pupils constrict to near stimuli but not light), and nystagmus.

Other choices and discussion

A. Bitemporal hemianopsia occurs with compression of the optic chiasm such as with a pituitary mass.
C. Seizures are not a component of Parinaud syndrome.
D. Ptosis, or drooping of the upper eyelid, is seen in Horner syndrome in contrast to eyelid retraction, which can be seen in Parinaud syndrome.
E. Internuclear ophthalmoplegia (INO) can occur in Parinaud syndrome but is less characteristic.

46.2 Correct: C. Diffuse midline glioma, H3 K27M-mutant.

Introduced in the 2016 updated version of the WHO classification of central nervous system (CNS) tumors, the diffuse midline glioma with H3 K27M mutation is an infiltrative, high-grade glioma in a midline or paramedian location that usually occurs in children. Typical locations are brainstem, thalamus, and cervical spinal cord.

Other choices and discussion

A. Medulloblastoma arises from the roof of the 4th ventricle, which is not demonstrated on the sagittal image shown here.
B. A glioblastoma is less common in children and typically presents as a heterogeneously enhancing and necrotic mass in the supratentorial brain.

D. A cavernous malformation would be expected to have a lobulated "popcorn" appearance and hypointense rim on T2-weighted imaging; this finding can be associated with a developmental venous anomaly.
E. Artery of Percheron infarct would present with signal abnormality of the bilateral paramedian thalami and/or midbrain, and not unilateral as seen in this case.

46.3 Correct: B. Imaging of the neuraxis is indicated.

Leptomeningeal spread and "brain-to-brain" metastases are common, and therefore imaging of the neuraxis is indicated on initial presentation.

Other choices and discussion

A. The enhancement pattern of H3 K27M-mutant gliomas is heterogeneous, although it is usually minimal or patchy and involves less than 25% of the tumor volume.
C. The H3 K27M mutation is associated with a worse prognosis in comparison to IDH-wildtype astrocytomas, with less than 10% of patients surviving for 2 years.
D. While H3 K27M-mutant gliomas most frequently occur in children, they can also occur in adults, making this answer choice incorrect.
E. H3 K27M-mutant gliomas have a poor prognosis with short overall survival; in contrast, tectal gliomas have an indolent course and most demonstrate stability over years.

References

Aboian MS, Solomon DA, Felton E, et al. Imaging characteristics of pediatric diffuse midline gliomas with histone H3 K27M mutation. *AJNR Am J Neuroradiol.* 2017;38(4):795–800.

Osborn AG. Diffuse Midline Glioma, H3 K27M-Mutant. In: Osborn AG, Hedlund GL, editors. Osborn's Brain: Imaging, Pathology, and Anatomy. 2nd ed. Philadelphia: Elsevier; 2018: 548–550.

Case 47

Please refer to the following images to answer the next three questions:

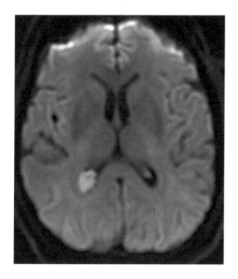 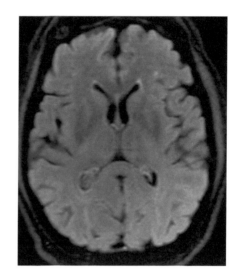

A 64-year-old male presents with generalized weakness.

47.1 What is the **MOST** likely diagnosis?

A. Xanthogranuloma.
B. Normal pressure hydrocephalus.
C. Creutzfeldt-Jakob disease.
D. Choroid plexus papilloma.
E. Epidermoid cyst.

47.2 What is the **MOST** common location?

A. Atrium of lateral ventricles.
B. Cerebral aqueduct.
C. Foramen of Monro.
D. Third ventricle.
E. Fourth ventricle.

47.3 What is the **BEST** next step in management?

A. Referral to neurosurgery for biopsy.
B. MRI in 6 months.
C. Obtain CT to evaluate for calcification.
D. No further action is necessary.
E. Obtain contrast-enhanced MRI.

Answers and Explanations

47.1 Correct: A. Xanthogranuloma.

Xanthogranuloma is a benign degenerative cystic mass, which is a common incidental finding in the choroid plexus in adults. Prevalence of xanthogranuloma increases with age. Most are bilateral, but unilateral xanthogranulomas are not infrequently seen. Most appear very hyperintense on diffusion-weighted imaging (DWI) and are incompletely suppressed on fluid-attenuated inversion recovery (FLAIR) as seen in this case.

Other choices and discussion

B. Disproportionate ventricular enlargement, not seen here, is typical of normal pressure hydrocephalus.
C. Cortical ribboning on DWI is expected in Creutzfeldt-Jakob disease.
D. Most choroid plexus papillomas in the lateral ventricle occur in children, not in older adults.
E. Although epidermoid cysts also demonstrate hyperintensity on DWI, this entity is not usually found in the atrium of the lateral ventricle.

47.2 Correct: A. Atrium of lateral ventricles.

The most common location is the atrium of the lateral ventricles.

Other choices and discussion

C–E. Less common locations are the third ventricle (**D**), fourth ventricle (**E**), and foramen of Monro (**C**). In these locations, however, there is the potential for obstructive hydrocephalus.

B. In these locations, however, there is the potential for obstructive hydrocephalus. Xanthogranulomas do not occur in the cerebral aqueduct.

47.3 Correct: D. No further action is necessary.

Xanthogranulomas are common incidental findings which are almost always of no clinical significance; therefore, no further action is needed.

Other choices and discussion

E, B. There is no need to evaluate for enhancement (**E**) or to obtain follow-up imaging (**B**); this benign lesion is of high-prevalence in the adult population.
A, C. Biopsy (**A**) is not indicated. There are often associated calcifications; however, there is no need to demonstrate this on CT in order to make the diagnosis (**C**).

References

Kinoshita T1, Moritani T, Hiwatashi A, et al. Clinically silent choroid plexus cyst: evaluation by diffusion-weighted MRI. *Neuroradiology.* 2005;47(4):251–255.

Pear BL. Xanthogranuloma of the choroid plexus. *AJR Am J Roentgenol.* 1984;143(2):401–402.

Case 48

Please refer to the following images to answer the next three questions:

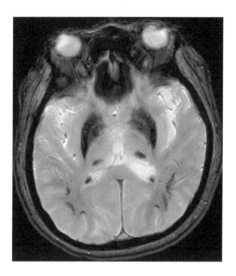
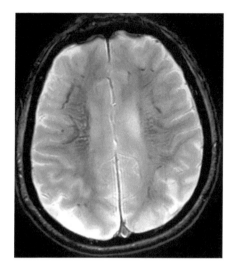

A 44-year-old otherwise healthy female presents with cognitive decline.

48.1 What is the **MOST** likely diagnosis?

A. Mineralizing microangiopathy.

B. Physiologic basal ganglia calcification.

C. Wilson disease.

D. Cerebral amyloid angiopathy.

E. Fahr disease.

48.2 Which of the following is associated with this diagnosis?

A. Diabetes mellitus.

B. Hyperparathyroidism.

C. Parkinsonism.

D. Alzheimer's dementia.

E. Frontotemporal dementia.

48.3 What is the **MOST** common site for this diagnosis?

A. Globus pallidus.

B. Dentate nucleus.

C. Cerebral white matter.

D. Pulvinar.

E. Putamen.

Answers and Explanations

48.1 Correct: E. Fahr disease.

In addition to a blooming hypointense signal in the basal ganglia on the gradient echo (GRE) image, involvement of the pulvinar nuclei of the thalami and subcortical white matter are also present here, rendering Fahr disease as the most likely diagnosis. Fahr disease, also known as primary familial brain calcification, demonstrates heavy, symmetric, and bilateral basal ganglia calcification, as seen in this patient.

Other choices and discussion

B. Physiologic, or senescent, basal ganglia calcification is milder, occurs in the medial (rather than lateral) globus pallidi, and presents in older adults who are at least 50 years old.
A. Mineralizing microangiopathy can appear similar to Fahr disease; however, this represents the long-term sequelae of whole brain irradiation.
C. Wilson disease presents with T2 hyperintensity in the putamen, globus pallidus, caudate, and ventrolateral thalamus (rather than pulvinar), which is not present in this case.
D. Cerebral amyloid angiopathy presents with several peripherally-located microhemorrhages in older patients (typically over 60 years old).

48.2 Correct: C. Parkinsonism.

Patients with Fahr disease are afflicted with insidious onset and progressive worsening of Parkinsonism, psychosis, and subcortical dementia. Although mineral deposition begins earlier, the clinical syndrome presents between ages 30 and 60.

Other choices and discussion

A. Diabetes mellitus is neither a cause nor an effect of Fahr disease.
B. Parathyroid hormone levels are normal, distinguishing patients with Fahr disease from hyperparathyroidism; the latter can present with a similar pattern of calcification on imaging.
D, E. There is no association with Alzheimer's or frontotemporal dementia.

48.3 Correct: A. Globus pallidus.

The most common location of calcification in Fahr disease is the globus pallidus, with lateral more characteristic than medial involvement.

Other choices and discussion

B–E. Additional although less common sites of involvement are the dentate nucleus of the cerebellum (**B**), cerebral white matter (**C**), pulvinar nucleus of the thalamus (**D**), caudate, and putamen (**E**).

References

Hegde AN, Mohan S, Lath N, et al. Differential diagnosis for bilateral abnormalities of the basal ganglia and thalamus. *Radiographics*. 2011;31:5–30.

Osborn AG. Primary Familial Brain Calcification. In: Osborn AG, Hedlund GL, editors. Osborn's Brain: Imaging, Pathology, and Anatomy. 2nd ed. Philadelphia: Elsevier; 2018: 1044–1047.

Case 49

Please refer to the following images to answer the next three questions:

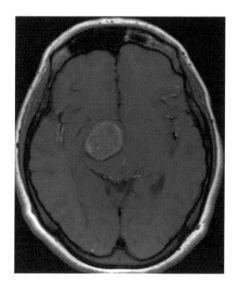
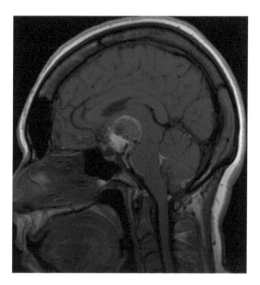

A 30-year-old female presents with sudden onset of seizures.

49.1 What is the **MOST** likely diagnosis?

A. Ruptured dermoid cyst.
B. Craniopharyngioma.
C. Epidermoid cyst.
D. Subarachnoid hemorrhage.
E. Lipoma.

49.2 What is the **MOST** common site for this diagnosis?

A. Cerebellopontine angle.
B. Fourth ventricle.
C. Suprasellar cistern.
D. Posterior fossa.
E. Frontonasal region.

49.3 Which of the following is **TRUE**?

A. Dermoid cysts are extra-axial lesions occurring off midline in location.
B. Epidermoids are less common than dermoid cysts.
C. Radiation is the treatment of choice if cyst is enlarging.
D. There is an association between cyst rupture and head trauma.
E. There is a high-rate of malignant transformation to squamous cell carcinoma.

Answers and Explanations

49.1 Correct: A. Ruptured dermoid cyst.

The axial and sagittal T1-weighted images show a large heterogeneous mass in the right suprasellar cistern, with intrinsic T1 hyperintensity consistent with fat. There is mass effect on the adjacent cerebral hemisphere, midbrain, and thalamus. There is also extensive intrinsic T1 hyperintensity within the subarachnoid spaces along the surface of the brain, which is consistent with diffusely dispersed fat. Imaging findings are most consistent with a ruptured dermoid cyst.

Other choices and discussion

C. Dermoid cysts follow fat on both CT and MRI sequences; in contrast, an epidermoid cyst follows cerebrospinal fluid (CSF) on imaging.
B. Craniopharyngioma also favors a suprasellar midline location, which is similar to dermoid cysts; however, this entity would be expected to be hypointense on T1-weighted imaging unless calcification or hemorrhage is present.
E. Lipomas are intrinsically T1 hyperintense; however, the signal is typically more homogeneous across the lesion than seen in this case.
D. Subarachnoid hemorrhage can present with intrinsic T1 hyperintensity in the subarachnoid spaces; however, this does not account for the large suprasellar mass on the images.

49.2 Correct: C. Suprasellar cistern.

Dermoid cysts are usually midline in location. The suprasellar cistern is the most common location.

Other choices and discussion

D, E. The posterior fossa **(D)** and then the frontonasal region **(E)** are the next common locations.
A. The fourth ventricle is not a typical location for dermoids.
B. The cerebellopontine angle is the most common location for epidermoid cysts, not dermoid cysts.

49.3 Correct: D. There is an association between cyst rupture and head trauma.

Cyst rupture can be spontaneous, especially in the setting of increasing size but can also be seen after head trauma.

Other choices and discussion

A. Dermoid cysts are extra-axial lesions; however, they tend to favor midline locations in contrast to epidermoid cysts which favor off-midline locations.
B. Epidermoid cysts are much more common than dermoid cysts; in fact, dermoid cysts account for less than 0.5% of all intracranial masses.
C. Surgical excision is the treatment of choice for dermoid cysts.
E. Complication by squamous cell carcinoma does occur with dermoid cysts, but it is rare.

References

Osborn AG, Preece MT. Intracranial cysts: radiologic-pathologic correlation and imaging approach. *Radiology*. 2006;239(3):650–664.

Ray MJ, Barnett DW, Snipes GJ, et al. Ruptured intracranial dermoid cyst. *Proceedings*. 2012;25(1):23–25.

Case 50

Please refer to the following images to answer the next three questions:

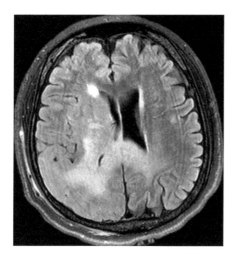 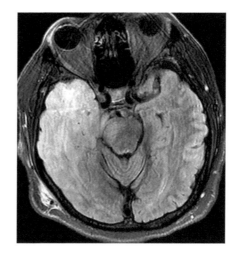

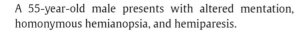

A 55-year-old male presents with altered mentation, homonymous hemianopsia, and hemiparesis.

50.1 What is the **MOST** likely diagnosis?

A. Progressive multifocal leukoencephalopathy (PML).

B. Metachromatic leukodystrophy (MLD).

C. Mitochondrial myopathy, encephalopathy, lactic acidosis, and stroke-like episodes (MELAS).

D. Diffuse midline glioma.

E. Gliomatosis spread of high-grade glioma.

50.2 Which of the following is **TRUE** of this diagnosis?

A. No longer considered a distinct entity in the WHO classification of central nervous system (CNS) tumors.

B. Histologic and clinical features are out of proportion to the imaging appearance.

C. Most cases are histologically classified as isocitrate dehydrogenase (IDH)-wild type glioblastoma (GBM).

D. Steroids are contraindicated.

E. Underlying brain architecture is destroyed.

50.3 How many lobes of involvement are required for this diagnosis?

A. 1.

B. 2.

C. 3.

D. 4.

E. No specific number of lobes, but bilateral involvement is required.

Answers and Explanations

50.1 Correct: E. Gliomatosis spread of high-grade glioma.

This pattern of high-grade glioma spread is not uncommonly misdiagnosed as a nonneoplastic white matter disease.

Other choices and discussion

A. PML demonstrates multifocal T2 and fluid-attenuated inversion recovery (FLAIR) hyperintense lesions; however, the characteristic predilection for subcortical U-fibers is absent in this case. In addition, in PML, there is usually an absence of mass effect on imaging and a history of an immunocompromised state.

B. Metachromatic leukodystrophy classically presents in toddlers, although there is also an adult form of the disease; in addition, the characteristic "butterfly" pattern of hemispheric white matter involvement is not observed here.

C. MELAS also presents with multifocal lesions; however, they are frequently cortical in location, unlike in this case.

D. Diffuse midline glioma is most commonly a pediatric tumor that involves the central brain structures such as the brainstem and thalami and unlikely in this middle-aged male.

50.2 Correct: A. No longer considered a distinct entity in the WHO classification of central nervous system (CNS) tumors.

Gliomatosis cerebri is no longer considered a distinct entity as of the 2016 updated version of the WHO classification of CNS tumors. The diagnosis is based on MRI appearance; however, the distinction does not bear any prognostic relevance, and tumors of varying histologic and molecular profiles can demonstrate the gliomatosis pattern of spread.

Other choices and discussion

B. The imaging appearance is typically out of proportion to the histologic and clinical features (i.e., the scans look worse than the patient).

C. Most tumors with gliomatosis pattern of spread on imaging are IDH-wild-type anaplastic astrocytomas, not GBM.

D. Steroids may help in the treatment of tumors exhibiting this pattern.

E. Despite the extensive infiltration and expansion of the involved white matter, the underlying cerebral architecture is grossly preserved.

50.3 Correct: C. 3.

Three lobes of involvement are required to meet the criteria for gliomatosis cerebri pattern.

Other choices and discussion

A, B, D. These are either less or more than the requisite number.

E. Involvement is frequently bilateral, although bilaterality is not required.

References

Herrlinger U, Jones DTW, Glas M, et al. Gliomatosis cerebri: no evidence for a separate brain tumor entity. *Acta Neuropathol.* 2016;131(2):309–319.

Morales La Madrid A, Ranjan S, Warren KE. Gliomatosis cerebri: a consensus summary report from the Second International Gliomatosis cerebri Group Meeting, June 22–23, 2017, Bethesda, USA. *J Neurooncol.* 2018;140(1):1–4.

Case 51

Challenge

Please refer to the following images to answer the next three questions:

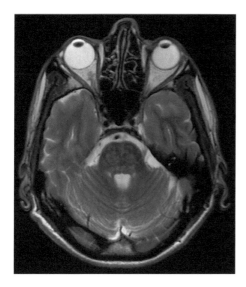 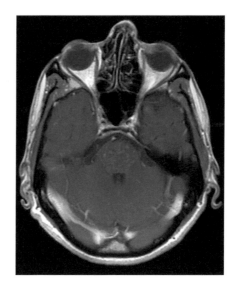

A 52-year-old male presents with progressive spastic quadriparesis.

51.1 What is the **BEST** next step in management?

A. Radiation therapy.

B. Lumbar puncture.

C. Cerebral angiogram.

D. Computed tomography (CT) chest, abdomen, and pelvis.

E. Biopsy.

51.2 The patient was started on steroids with rapid clinical and radiological improvement. Clinical workup did not reveal a specific diagnosis. What is the **MOST** likely diagnosis?

A. Neurosarcoidosis.

B. Diffuse midline glioma.

C. Vasculitis.

D. CLIPPERS.

E. Behçet's disease.

51.3 What imaging finding is **MOST** specific for CLIPPERS?

A. Punctate and curvilinear enhancing lesions in the pons and cerebellum without edema or mass effect.

B. Expansile, enhancing pontine mass.

C. Multiple T2 hyperintense lesions with leading edge of enhancement.

D. Rounded T2 hypointense lesions with nodular enhancement and surrounding edema.

E. Multiple punctate and linear foci of restricted diffusion with variable enhancement.

Answers and Explanations

51.1 Correct: B. Lumbar puncture.

Multiple enhancing lesions in the brainstem has a wide differential diagnosis, including neurosarcoidosis, metastasis, intravascular lymphoma, demyelination, infections such as tuberculosis and Whipple's disease, and chronic lymphocytic inflammation with pontine perivascular enhancement responsive to steroids (CLIPPERS). Lumbar puncture should be obtained initially to look for an inflammatory or neoplastic cerebrospinal fluid (CSF) profile, microbiologic studies, and cytology.

Other choices and discussion

A. Radiation therapy is an important therapy in metastasis and glioma; however, this would not likely be pursued prior to a more certain diagnosis.
C. Cerebral angiogram is helpful in assessing for vasculitis, but would be considered after lumbar puncture.
D. CT of the chest, abdomen, and pelvis may be indicated to assess for a primary malignancy or extra-CNS involvement of sarcoidosis but should follow a lumbar puncture.
E. Biopsy of the brainstem is a relatively high-risk and invasive procedure, and is not the first diagnostic procedure to pursue.

51.2 Correct: D. CLIPPERS.

Chronic lymphocytic inflammation with pontine perivascular enhancement responsive to steroids (CLIPPERS) is an encephalomyelitis which predominately involves the brainstem, most commonly the pons. Pathologically, brain biopsy shows a perivascular CD3 + T cell predominant lymphocytic inflammation. On imaging, there are small nodular and curvilinear enhancing lesions in the brainstem, with relatively mild T2 signal compared with the enhancement, and without significant surrounding edema. While these imaging features are suggestive of CLIPPERS, they are not specific, and a wide differential should be initially considered as detailed in question 1. The diagnosis may be made by brain biopsy, or clinically if the patient responds appropriately to steroids and other diagnoses are excluded.

Other choices and discussion

A. Neurosarcoidosis may also have nodular enhancing parenchymal lesions similar to CLIPPERS, although isolated central nervous system (CNS) involvement of sarcoidosis is uncommon. Patients with sarcoidosis may also have elevated serum angiotensin converting enzyme (ACE) levels.
B. Diffuse midline glioma typically presents as a mass-like lesion with T2 FLAIR hyperintense signal within the thalami or brainstem. The enhancement pattern is variable. The absence of a mass-like lesion in conjunction with rapid clinical and radiological improvement following steroids makes this a less likely diagnosis.
C. Brainstem lesions from vasculitis are related to infarcts which will enhance if subacute, and diagnosis is made on vascular imaging with computed tomography angiography (CTA), MRI or digital subtraction angiography (DSA).
E. Behçet's disease is a systemic inflammatory disorder resulting in oral and genital ulcers, and may involve the CNS with T2 hyperintense lesions, patchy enhancement, and surrounding edema in the brainstem and thalamus.

51.3 Correct: A. Punctate and curvilinear enhancing lesions in the pons and cerebellum without edema or mass effect.

CLIPPERS is an encephalomyelitis which predominately involves the brainstem. "MRI" findings of curvilinear and nodular enhancing lesions in the pons and cerebellum with mild T2 signal and without surrounding edema should raise the possibility of CLIPPERS. The diagnosis of CLIPPERS is made if the patient responds to steroid treatment and alternative diagnoses are excluded.

Other choices and discussion

B. An expansile, enhancing pontine mass is not specific for CLIPPERS, but glioma, lymphoma, and metastasis should be considered.
C. Multiple T2 hyperintense lesions with a leading edge of enhancement are seen with demyelination.
D. Rounded T2 hypointense lesions with nodular enhancement and surrounding edema are concerning for tuberculous or fungal infection.
E. Multiple punctate and linear foci of restricted diffusion with variable enhancement are typical of acute and subacute infarcts, and vascular imaging to assess for vasculitis, dissection, and embolic source should be obtained.

References

Pittock SJ, Debruyne J, Krecke KN, et al. Chronic lymphocytic inflammation with pontine perivascular enhancement responsive to steroids (CLIPPERS). *Brain.* 2010;133(9):2626–2634.

Zalewski NL, Tobin WO. CLIPPERS. *Curr Neurol Neurosci Rep.* 2017;17(9):65.

Case 52

Challenge

Please refer to the following images to answer the next three questions:

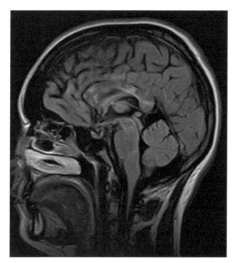

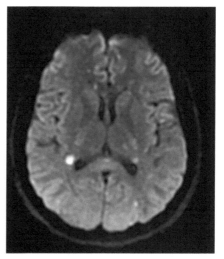

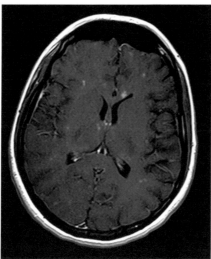

A 25-year-old female, with a history of systemic lupus erythematosus and polysubstance abuse, presents with progressive confusion and memory loss.

52.1 What is the **MOST** likely diagnosis?

A. Septic emboli.

B. Primary angiitis of the central nervous system (CNS).

C. Multiple sclerosis.

D. Levamisole toxicity.

E. Susac syndrome.

52.2 What test will confirm the diagnosis?

A. Fluoroscein retinal angiography.

B. Lumbar puncture.

C. Cerebral angiography.

D. Serum toxicology screen.

E. Echocardiography.

52.3 What is the classic clinical triad of Susac syndrome?

A. Confusion, ophthalmoplegia, and ataxia.

B. Dementia, urinary incontinence, and gait abnormality.

C. Encephalopathy, hearing loss, and branch retinal artery occlusions.

D. Periorbital pain, cranial nerve VI palsy, and otitis media.

E. Hypertension, bradycardia, and irregular breathing.

Answers and Explanations

52.1 Correct: E. Susac syndrome.

Susac syndrome, also known as retinocochleocerebral vasculopathy or SICRET syndrome (small infarctions of cochlear, retinal, and encephalic tissue), is a rare disorder of the small arteries of the brain, retina, and inner ear. It is likely autoimmune in etiology, usually affecting women in their third and fourth decades. It shows characteristic findings on "MRI", with small, rounded T2 hyperintense lesions in the central corpus callosum as well as additional small lesions in the white matter related to small infarcts. Lesions may show restricted diffusion if acute or enhancement if subacute.

Other choices and discussion
C. Because Susac syndrome is rare, usually affects young women, and has white matter lesions involving the corpus callosum, it may be misdiagnosed as multiple sclerosis (MS). It is important to distinguish between the two entities: MS lesions are larger, ovoid and perivenular in orientation, and involve the callosalseptal interface rather than the central corpus callosum.
A. Septic emboli may also show multiple small infarcts; however, they are in the border zone distribution and will not preferentially involve the corpus callosum.
B. Primary angiitis of the CNS will also demonstrate multiple small infarcts of varying ages without preferential involvement of the corpus callosum.
D. Levamisole toxicity may occur in cocaine users who took cocaine adulterated with levamisole; these patients present with an acute inflammatory demyelination. Multiple ovoid, enhancing lesions are seen on MRI with levamisole toxicity and without involvement of the corpus callosum.

52.2 Correct: A. Fluorescein retinal angiography.

Fluorescein retinal angiography allows for visualization of branch retinal artery occlusions, a finding of Susac syndrome that would not be seen in the other differential considerations generated from MRI. Susac syndrome is likely autoimmune, and different autoantibodies are under investigation.

Other choices and discussion
B, D. Currently, no serum or cerebrospinal fluid (CSF) markers are part of the diagnostic workup, and lumbar puncture (**B**) or toxicology screen (**D**) cannot confirm the diagnosis.
C. The vessels involved are too small to be seen on cerebral angiography.
E. Echocardiography is important in the workup of cerebral emboli, but does not have a role in the evaluation of Susac syndrome.

52.3 Correct: C. Encephalopathy, hearing loss, and branch retinal artery occlusions.

Susac syndrome (also known as SICRET syndrome [small infarctions of cochlear, retinal, and encephalic tissue] or retinocochleocerebral vasculopathy) is a rare, likely autoimmune disorder with the classic clinical triad of encephalopathy, hearing loss, and branch retinal artery occlusions. It is important to note that some or all of these classic features may not be present in a given patient. Susac syndrome has classic imaging findings related to small infarcts of varying ages, and preferential involvement of the central corpus callosum. These infarcts will show restrict diffusion if acute, enhancement if subacute, and residual T2/fluid-attenuated inversion recovery (FLAIR) hyperintensity when chronic. When suspected, fluorescein retinal angiography should be obtained to assess for branch retinal artery occlusions.

Other choices and discussion
A. Confusion, ophthalmoplegia, and ataxia is the classic clinical triad of Wernicke's encephalopathy.
B. Dementia, urinary incontinence, and gait abnormality is the triad of normal pressure hydrocephalus; also known as "wet, wobbly, and wacky."
D. Periorbital pain, cranial nerve VI palsy, and otitis media is Gradenigo's triad, which is seen in petrous apicitis.
E. Hypertension, bradycardia, and irregular breathing is Cushing's triad, secondary to intracranial hypertension.

References

Do TH, Fisch C, Evoy F. Susac syndrome: report of four cases and review of the literature. *AJNR Am J Neuroradiol.* 2004;25(3):382–388.
Saenz R, Quan AW, Magalhaes A, et al. MRI of Susac's syndrome. *AJR Am J Roentgenol.* 2005;184(5):1688–1690.

Case 53

Challenge

Please refer to the following images to answer the next three questions:

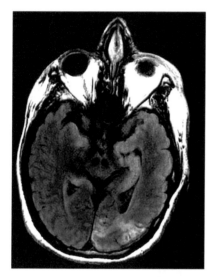

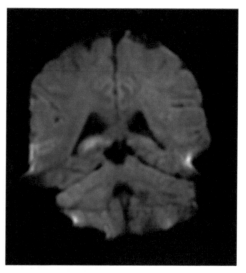

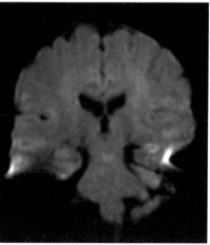

A 52-year-old male with history of myelodysplastic syndrome status post bone marrow transplantation presents with worsening altered mental status.

53.1 What is the **BEST** next step in management?

A. Stroke workup.

B. Lumbar puncture.

C. Antibiotics.

D. Thiamine repletion.

E. Biopsy.

53.2 What is the **MOST** likely diagnosis?

A. Transient global amnesia.

B. Wernicke's encephalopathy.

C. Diffuse infiltrative glioma.

D. Infectious encephalitis.

E. Seizure related changes.

53.3 What is the primary risk factor for Human herpesvirus 6 (HHV-6) encephalitis?

A. Organ transplantation (solid organ or stem cell).

B. Travel history to endemic area.

C. Nosocomial exposure.

D. Congenital immunodeficiency syndromes.

E. IV drug use.

Answers and Explanations

53.1 Correct: B. Lumbar puncture.

MRI shows increased fluid-attenuated inversion recovery (FLAIR) signal and restricted diffusion in the bilateral mesial temporal lobes. The primary differential considerations are viral encephalitides, specifically herpes simplex virus (HSV1/2) and human herpesvirus 6 (HHV-6) as well as autoimmune encephalitis. Lumbar puncture is the next appropriate step to assess for HSV and HHV-6 in cerebrospinal fluid (CSF) as well as autoimmune antibodies.

Other choices and discussion

A. The bilateral restricted diffusion is not in a vascular distribution, and stroke workup is not necessary.
C. The bilateral pattern is not typical of bacterial encephalitis, and empiric antibiotics would be held prior to lumbar puncture.
D. Thiamine repletion is the treatment in Wernicke's encephalopathy, which manifests as FLAIR and diffusion-weighted imaging (DWI) signal in the mammillary bodies, medial thalami, and periaqueductal grey matter. The mesial temporal lobes are spared in Wernicke's encephalopathy.
E. Biopsy is not indicated initially and may be considered if workup is negative and/or if the signal abnormality progresses.

53.2 Correct: D. Infectious encephalitis.

The top consideration is a viral encephalitis, with bilateral FLAIR signal and restricted diffusion in the bilateral mesial temporal lobes, and immunosuppressed status after bone marrow transplantation, specifically HSV and HHV-6.

Other choices and discussion

A. Transient global amnesia can show punctate foci of restricted diffusion in the hippocampi (<3 mm), rather than the diffuse restricted diffusion in the hippocampi in this case. Patients with transient global amnesia will also have a classic clinical syndrome of acute onset of memory loss with resolution in approximately 24 hours.
B. Wernicke's encephalopathy occurs due to thiamine deficiency, with MRI showing increased T2/FLAIR signal in the mammillary bodies, medial thalami, periaqueductal grey, and tectum of the midbrain. Diffusion restriction and enhancement may also be present in the affected regions. The mesial temporal lobes are typically spared.

C. Diffuse infiltrative glioma may mimic a viral encephalitis when primarily affecting the mesial temporal lobe, but is not a likely consideration in this case given the bilaterally of signal abnormality and lack of associated expansion.
E. Seizures if prolonged and uncontrolled can cause T2/FLAIR signal and diffusion restriction in the hippocampi. It is less likely in this case, as seizure changes are typically unilateral, affecting the hemisphere with the ictal focus.

53.3 Correct: A. Organ transplantation (solid organ or stem cell).

Human herpesvirus 6 (HHV-6) is a common virus to which >90% of the population is exposed by 2 years of age, with initial exposure asymptomatic or causing roseola infantum and exanthem subitum. In immunocompromised patients, the latent virus can cause a severe encephalitis. Patients who have undergone solid organ or stem cell transplantation and are immunosuppressed are at greatest risk of HHV-6 encephalitis, which manifests on MRI as transient bilateral mesial temporal T2/FLAIR signal abnormality and restricted diffusion. This overlaps with herpes simplex virus (HSV) encephalitis. Helpful distinguishing features are extratemporal involvement, which is more common with HSV encephalitis than with HHV-6 encephalitis, and the transient nature of the signal abnormality in HHV-6 encephalitis versus HSV encephalitis; in the latter, the signal typically persists for a longer period of time.

Other choices and discussion

B, C, E. As the majority of the population is exposed as a child and has latent virus, further exposure is not a primary risk factor.
D. While any immunocompromised patient is at increased risk of HHV-6 encephalitis, it is mostly seen in patients who have solid organ or stem cell transplantation.

References

Noguchi T, Mihara F, Yoshiura T, et al. MR imaging of human herpesvirus-6 encephalopathy after hematopoietic stem cell transplantation in adults. *AJNR Am J Neuroradiol.* 2006;27(10):2191-2195.
Noguchi T, Yoshiura T, Hiwatashi A, et al. CT and MRI findings of human herpesvirus 6-associated encephalopathy: comparison with findings of herpes simplex virus encephalitis. *AJR Am J Roentgenol.* 2010;194(3):754–760.

Case 54

Challenge

Please refer to the following images to answer the next three questions:

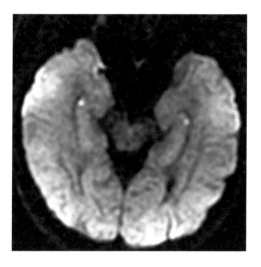
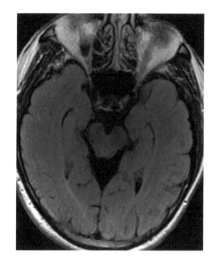

A 58-year-old female with acute memory loss.

54.1 What is the **MOST** likely diagnosis?

A. Nonconvulsive status epilepticus.

B. Transient global amnesia.

C. Wernicke's encephalopathy.

D. HSV encephalitis.

E. Migraine.

54.2 What is the **BEST** next step in management?

A. Electroencephalogram (EEG).

B. Lumbar puncture.

C. Digital subtraction angiography (DSA).

D. MRI follow-up at 3 months.

E. Reassurance.

54.3 What is the typical imaging finding of TGA?

A. Punctate foci of DWI hyperintensity in the hippocampus.

B. T2 hyperintensity in the medial thalami, hypothalamus, mamillary bodies, and periaqueductal grey matter.

C. Diffuse unilateral hippocampal DWI hyperintensity and swelling.

D. Asymmetric bilateral temporal cortical T2 hyperintensity and swelling.

E. Small foci of DWI hyperintensity in the corpus callosum.

Answers and Explanations

54.1 Correct: B. Transient global amnesia.

Punctate foci of diffusion-weighted imaging (DWI) hyperintensity are present in both hippocampi without corresponding T2/fluid-attenuated inversion recovery (FLAIR) signal abnormality or enhancement, which are classic findings of transient global amnesia (TGA).

Other choices and discussion

A. The MRI changes related to status epilepticus include hippocampal DWI signal abnormality, which involves the entire hippocampal formation with swelling related to cytotoxic edema.

C. Hippocampal signal abnormality is not typical of Wernicke's encephalopathy, which involves the medial thalami, hypothalamus, mamillary bodies, and periaqueductal grey matter.

D. HSV encephalitis typically has asymmetric bilateral temporal cortical T2 signal abnormality. The hippocampus may be involved; however, the extent of signal abnormality is far more extensive.

E. Acute migraine typically shows no abnormality on routine MRI. Perfusion abnormalities may be seen in an acute phase. Chronic migraines show increased T2 hyperintense foci in the subcortical white matter, which are often difficult to differentiate from other causes of chronic small vessel disease.

54.2 Correct: E. Reassurance.

If the clinical syndrome is clear, the course of TGA is self-limited and does not require further workup or follow-up. All other choices are incorrect.

Other choices and discussion

A–D. These answer choices are not indicated in classic TGA, which is often transient and does not require further diagnostic work-up.

54.3 Correct: A. Punctate foci of DWI hyperintensity in the hippocampus.

Small (<3 mm) DWI hyperintense lesion(s) in the hippocampus are the classic findings in TGA. The etiology of these lesions is uncertain. MRI may also be normal in TGA; however, high-field strength and b-value may improve detection of these small lesions. They resolve completely on follow-up imaging.

Other choices and discussion

B. T2 hyperintensity in the medial thalami, hypothalamus, mamillary bodies, and periaqueductal grey matter is typical of Wernicke's encephalopathy.

C. Diffuse unilateral hippocampal DWI hyperintensity and swelling is a finding associated with cytotoxic edema from status epilepticus.

D. Asymmetric bilateral temporal cortical T2 hyperintensity and swelling is typical of HSV encephalitis. Hemorrhage is also often present.

E. Small foci of DWI hyperintensity in the corpus callosum is suggestive of Susac syndrome or retinocochleocerebral vasculopathy, which in addition to callosal involvement has numerous small infarcts or T2 hyperintense lesions in the periventricular white matter, internal capsule, and brainstem.

References

Hunter G. Transient global amnesia. *Neurol Clin.* 2011;29(4):1045–1054.

Weon YC, Kim JH, Lee JS, et al. Optimal diffusion-weighted imaging protocol for lesion detection in transient global amnesia. *AJNR Am J Neuroradiol.* 2008;29(7):1324–1328.

Case 55

Challenge

Please refer to the following images to answer the next three questions:

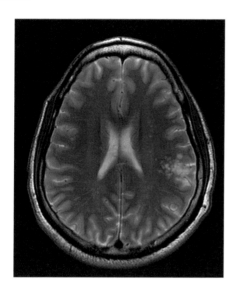 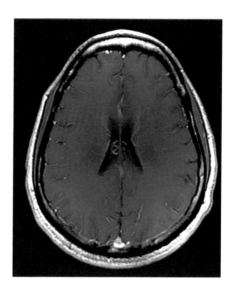

A 47-year-old male with chronic headaches.

55.1 What is the **MOST** likely diagnosis?

A. Multinodular and vacuolating neuronal tumor (MVNT).

B. Dysembryoplastic neuroepithelial tumor (DNET).

C. Tumefactive perivascular spaces.

D. Diffuse infiltrative astrocytoma.

E. Cryptococcal infection.

55.2 What is the **BEST** next step in management?

A. Biopsy.

B. Resection.

C. Reassurance.

D. Electroencephalogram (EEG).

E. Lumbar puncture.

55.3 Which part of the brain is **MOST** commonly affected in MVNT?

A. Cerebral hemispheres.

B. Basal ganglia.

C. Cerebellar hemispheres.

D. Pons.

E. Midbrain.

Answers and Explanations

55.1 Correct: A. Multinodular and vacuolating neuronal tumor (MVNT).

MVNT is a rare benign lesion with characteristic imaging featuresa—cluster of small rounded T2 and fluid-attenuated inversion recovery (FLAIR) hyperintense foci in the subcortical white matter of the cerebrum, without enhancement, mass effect, or edema. It is usually incidentally found in patients in their 4th and 5th decades. The association with seizures is currently uncertain. While it has been reported as epileptogenic in some case reports, many patients with MVNT do not experience seizures.

Other choices and discussion

B. DNET is also a "bubbly" lesion with multiple T2 hyperintense foci; however, these foci are not discontinuous as they are in MVNT. The temporal lobe is most commonly affected, and patients usually present in childhood with seizures associated with DNET.

C. Tumefactive perivascular spaces are multiple dilated perivascular spaces identifiable by their tubular morphology, radial orientation, and suppression of T2 signal on FLAIR. As their name suggests, they can have mass effect and surrounding edema or gliosis.

D. Infiltrative astrocytoma is an ill-defined and expansile mass with T2 signal abnormality.

E. Cryptococcal central nervous system (CNS) infection may result in gelatinous pseudocysts, irregular rounded T2 hyperintense cystic lesions along perivascular spaces, often involving the inferior basal ganglia. Edema and parenchymal or leptomeningeal enhancement can be seen with cryptococcal meningitis.

55.2 Correct: C. Reassurance.

MVNT is a benign lesion which does not require follow-up if the diagnosis is clear.

Other choices and discussion

A, B. MVNT should not be biopsied (**A**) or resected (**B**) unless it is thought to be a seizure focus.

D. An EEG would be warranted if the patient experiences seizures but not if MVNT is discovered incidentally.

E. Lumbar puncture does not have a role in the diagnosis of MVNT.

55.3 Correct: A. Cerebral hemispheres.

MVNT is a newly defined benign lesion with characteristic imaging features. MVNT is typically incidental, although potentially epileptogenic if the patient experiences seizures. It demonstrates multiple small discontinuous T2 hyperintense foci in the subcortical white matter of the cerebrum. There is no associated enhancement, mass effect, or edema. It has been reported most commonly in the supratentorial cerebrum.

Other choices and discussion

C. MVNTs have been reported in the cerebellar hemispheres but to a much lesser degree than in the supratentorial cerebral hemispheres.

B, D–E. MVNTs have not been reported in the basal ganglia or brainstem (medulla, pons, and midbrain).

References

Kapucu I, Jhaveri MD, Kocak M, et al. Multinodular and Vacuolating Neuronal Tumor of the Cerebrum: A Benign Nonaggressive Cerebral Lesion. *Eur Neurol.* 2018;79(1-2): 74–75.

Nunes RH, Hsu CC, da Rocha AJ, et al. Multinodular and Vacuolating Neuronal Tumor of the Cerebrum: A New "Leave Me Alone" Lesion with a Characteristic Imaging Pattern. *AJNR Am J Neuroradiol.* 2017;38(10):1899–1904.

Case 56

Challenge

Please refer to the following images to answer the next three questions:

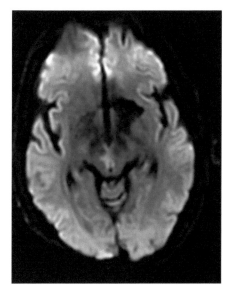
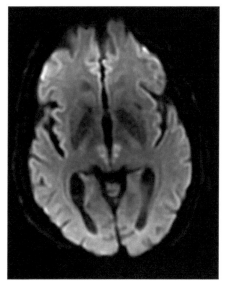
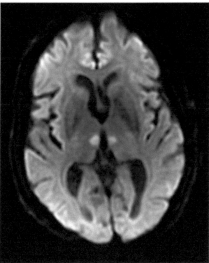

A 92-year-old male presents with altered mental status.

56.1 What is the **MOST** likely diagnosis?

A. Wernicke's encephalopathy.
B. Deep venous sinus thrombosis.
C. Creutzfeldt Jakob disease (CJD).
D. Carbon monoxide poisoning.
E. Artery of Percheron infarct.

56.2 What is the **BEST** next step in management?

A. Stroke workup with echocardiogram to assess for embolic source.

B. Cerebral angiography and thrombectomy.
C. Lumbar puncture.
D. Biopsy.
E. Vessel wall imaging.

56.3 Which artery does the artery of Percheron arise from?

A. Basilar artery.
B. Superior cerebellar artery.
C. Posterior communicating artery.
D. P1 segment of the posterior cerebral artery.
E. P2 segment of the posterior cerebral artery.

Answers and Explanations

56.1 Correct: E. Artery of Percheron infarct.

There is restricted diffusion in the central midbrain and ventromedial thalami, in the territory of the variant artery of Percheron, consistent with acute infarct.

Other choices and discussion

A. Wernicke's encephalopathy involves similar regions with T2/fluid-attenuated inversion recovery (FLAIR) signal abnormality and variable restricted diffusion, but the signal abnormality extends beyond the territory of the artery of Percheron to the dorsal thalami and the mamillary bodies.

B. Deep venous thrombosis of the internal cerebral veins, vein of Galen, or straight sinus, may result in venous infarcts in the thalami. However, there is typically more extensive involvement of the thalami, with swelling from venous congestion and possibly hemorrhage.

C. CJD is a spongiform encephalopathy with variable restricted diffusion involving the cerebral cortex, basal ganglia, and thalami. Thalamic involvement of CJD is in the pulvinar and dorsomedial regions.

D. Carbon monoxide poisoning results in hypoxic cerebral injury, most commonly manifesting as restricted diffusion in the bilateral globus palladi.

56.2 Correct: A. Stroke workup with echocardiogram to assess for embolic source.

Artery of Percheron infarct results from arterial occlusion by thromboembolism or in situ arterial thrombosis, and requires a stroke workup for the assessment of thromboembolic sources and risk factors of atherosclerotic disease.

Other choices and discussion

B. Tissue plasminogen activator (tPA) may be administered as per clinical guidelines, if within the appropriate window, but an occluded artery of Percheron is too small to be treated by mechanical thrombectomy.

C. Lumbar puncture is not part of the routine stroke workup, although it plays a role if there is concern for vasculitis as a cause of the infarct.

D. There is no role for biopsy.

E. Vessel wall imaging may play a role in the workup of vasculitis and cryptogenic stroke but does not currently have a role in routine stroke workup.

56.3 Correct: D. P1 segment of the posterior cerebral artery.

The artery of Percheron is a rare but important anatomic variant. It arises from the P1 segment and supplies both medial thalami, in place of the more common bilateral medial thalamic perforators. Occlusion of the artery of Percheron results in infarction of the bilateral medial thalami, with variable involvement of the midbrain. Prognosis depends on midbrain involvement, with better prognosis if the midbrain is spared. The incidence of this variant anatomy is unknown. It is important to differentiate this arterial variation from normal vascular territories for accurate stroke diagnosis.

Other choices and discussion

A, B, C, E. These answer choices are incorrect because the artery of Percheron arises from the P1 segment of the posterior cerebral artery.

References

Arauz A, Patiño-Rodríguez HM, Vargas-González JC, et al. Clinical spectrum of artery of Percheron infarct: clinical-radiological correlations. *J Stroke Cerebrovasc Dis.* 2014;23(5):1083–1088.

Krampla W, Schmidbauer B, Hruby W. Ischaemic stroke of the artery of Percheron (2007: 10b). *Eur Radiol.* 2008;18(1):192–194.

Case 57

Challenge

Please refer to the following images to answer the next three questions:

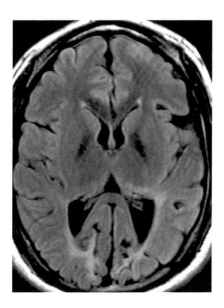 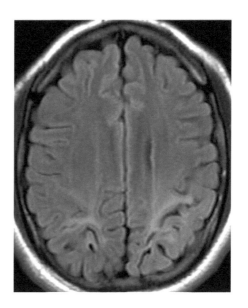

A 22-year-old male with history of developmental delay and seizure disorder since early childhood.

57.1 What is the **MOST** likely explanation for the imaging findings above?

A. Traumatic brain injury.

B. Congenital infection.

C. Bilateral posterior cerebral artery (PCA) infarction.

D. Neonatal hypoglycemic brain injury.

E. Posterior reversible encephalopathy syndrome (PRES).

57.2 Which of the following imaging findings is **MOST** predictive of a clinical hypoglycemic episode occurring in the setting of HIE?

A. Basal ganglia injury.

B. Cerebral watershed injury.

C. Posterior gray matter injury.

D. Posterior white matter and pulvinar injury.

E. Anteromedial thalamic injury.

57.3 What is the **MOST** common clinical manifestation of neonatal hypoglycemia?

A. Stupor or tremulousness.

B. Seizures.

C. Respiratory depression or apnea.

D. Irritability.

E. Hypotonia, inactivity, or apathy.

Answers and Explanations

57.1 Correct: D. Neonatal hypoglycemic brain injury.

In the above case, fluid-attenuated inversion recovery (FLAIR) images show bilateral and symmetric abnormally elevated signal intensity in the occipital and parietal white matter, associated with cortical thinning and enlargement of the occipital horns. The findings are typical for sequelae of prior neonatal hypoglycemic brain injury. Hypoglycemia can occur in newborns who are afflicted with asphyxia, newborns of diabetic mothers, and newborns who are of low birthweight for gestational age. Newborns symptomatic from hypoglycemia are at risk of permanent brain damage. Diffusion-weighted imaging (DWI) performed within 6 days of injury shows restricted diffusion in the occipital lobes. Diffusion restriction may also be seen in the thalamus, particularly in the pulvinar and the corpus callosum. DWI abnormalities may normalize if performed beyond this window. Patterns of injury on T1 and T2 sequences performed early in the postinjury period, but not necessarily within the 6-day window, show more diverse patterns of injuries including: global white matter injury, isolated periventricular white matter injury, isolated posterior white matter injury, basal ganglia and posterior limb of the internal capsule injuries, and cortical injuries.

Other choices and discussion

A. Focal parenchymal lesions in traumatic brain injury include contusions and axonal shear injuries, which do not fit the pattern demonstrated here.
B. Congenital infection results in various patterns of brain injuries that are dependent on the responsible pathogen, but parieto-occipital involvement is not one of them.
C. The pattern and morphologic characteristics of the injury in the question stem do not conform to what may be expected from bilateral PCA infarcts.
E. PRES manifests acutely on imaging as vasogenic edema in the cerebral watershed zones, with varying degrees of cortical, subcortical white matter, and deep white matter involvement. There is a predilection for the posterior watershed, although the frontal lobes can also be affected. While the findings in the question stem are parietal and occipital in location, there is also volume loss, indicating a chronic process. Abnormalities in PRES are also usually reversible, although PRES can be complicated by infarction and hemorrhage. No clues in the history supportive of PRES (such as hypertension or cyclosporine treatment) are provided.

57.2 Correct: D. Posterior white matter and pulvinar injury.

Neonatal encephalopathy (NE) refers to a disturbance in neurological function in the earliest days of life of a term infant. NE has many causes, the most common being HIE. Other causes include cerebral dysgenesis and congenital infection. Neonates with HIE are at risk of developing hypoglycemia and both patterns of injury may be present when neonates with NE are imaged (the standard of care is to image at day 3). Patterns of brain injury due to hypoglycemia can be varied. In the acute phase (within 6 days), restricted diffusion can be seen in the occipital lobes, thalami, and corpus callosum. In the early phase, but not necessarily within the first 6 days, variable patterns of injury in the white matter and basal ganglia on T1- and T2-weighted images can be seen. Posterior white matter and pulvinar injury (**D**) on DWI and/or T1- and T2-weighted imaging when performed in the acute phase, however, appear(s) to be most predictive of clinical hypoglycemia in the setting of clinical HIE either in the presence or absence of superimposed imaging findings of HIE.

Other choices and discussion

A, B. Basal ganglia injury and cerebral watershed injuries are involved in profound and prolonged partial asphyxia, respectively.
C, E. Posterior gray matter injury and anteromedial thalamic injury can be seen within the constellation of injuries resulting from HIE or hypoglycemia, but are not independently predictive of a clinical hypoglycemic episode.

57.3 Correct: A. Stupor or tremulousness.

Stupor and tremulousness are the most common clinical manifestations of neonatal hypoglycemia.

Other choices and discussion

B–E. Seizures (**B**), respiratory depression or apnea (**C**), irritability (**D**), and hypotonia, inactivity, or apathy (**E**) are less frequent clinical manifestations.

References

Barkovich AJ, Ali FA, Rowley HA, et al. Imaging Patterns of Neonatal Hypoglycemia. *AJNR Am J Neuroradiol.* 1998;19:523–528.

Bartynski WS. Posterior Reversible Encephalopathy Syndrome, Part 1: Fundamental Imaging and Clinical Features. *AJNR Am J Neuroradiol.* 2008;29(6):1036–1042.

Vannucci RC, Vannucci SJ. Hypoglycemic brain injury. *Seminars in Neonatology* 2001;6:147–155.

Wong DST, Poskitt KJ, Chau V, et al. Brain Injury Patterns in Hypoglycemia in Neonatal Encephalopathy. *AJNR Am J Neuroradiol.* 2013;34(7):1456–1461.

Case 58

Challenge

Please refer to the following images to answer the next three questions:

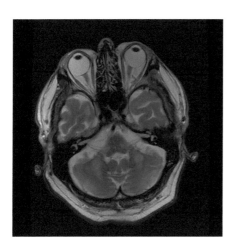 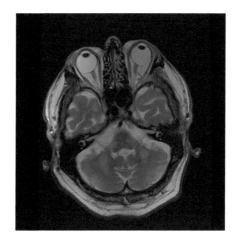

A 70-year-old male, with family history notable for siblings with mild learning disability, presents with cognitive decline and mild ataxia.

58.1 Which is the **MOST** likely diagnosis based on the history and imaging findings?

A. Vascular dementia.

B. Multiple sclerosis (MS).

C. Multiple system atrophy, cerebellar subtype (MSA-C).

D. Fragile-X-associated tremor/ataxia syndrome (FXTAS).

E. Parkinson's disease.

58.2 Which genetic abnormality is responsible for FXTAS?

A. Deletion of the *FMR1* gene.

B. Expansion of a trinucleotide repeat in the untranslated region of the *FMR1 gene.*

C. Methylation of the *FMR1* gene with resultant transcriptional silencing.

D. Missense mutation in the *FMR1* gene.

E. Deletion of the *FMR1* promoter.

58.3 What is the mode of inheritance for FXTAS?

A. Autosomal dominant pattern.

B. Autosomal recessive pattern.

C. X-linked dominant pattern.

D. X-linked recessive pattern.

E. Mitochondrial pattern.

Answers and Explanations

58.1 Correct: D. Fragile X-associated tremor/ataxia syndrome (FXTAS).

The T2-weighted images show increased signal in the middle cerebellar peduncles (MCPs) and the cerebellar white matter about the dentate nuclei as well as findings of cerebral and cerebellar atrophy. In the provided clinical context, findings are most consistent with FXTAS. FXTAS is a neurodegenerative disorder characterized by late-onset cognitive decline, cerebellar ataxia, and intention tremor. Males are more frequently affected than females. MRI features in FXTAS include increased T2 signal in the cerebellar white matter lateral, inferior, and superior to the dentate nuclei, with similar signal changes present in the middle cerebellar peduncles. Cerebellar and cerebral atrophy is present.

Other choices and discussion
A. Imaging findings in individuals with vascular dementia include multiple infarcts and changes of small vessel ischemic disease. The middle cerebellar peduncle (MCP) signal change, however, would be unusual in vascular dementia.
B. Demyelinating plaques of multiple sclerosis are found in the cortical/juxtacortical, periventricular, and infratentorial regions, but the vast majority of MS diagnoses are made in patients in the 20 to 50-year age range.
C. Imaging findings of MSA-C include cerebellar and pontine atrophy and signal abnormality in the MCPs. Absent in the above case, however, is the "hot-cross bun" sign—cruciate T2 signal abnormality in the pons related to degeneration of the pontine nuclei and pontocerebellar fibers—which is characteristic but not specific to MSA-C.
E. Parkinson's disease is a neurodegenerative movement disorder characterized by resting tremor, rigidity, and hypokinesia due to degeneration of dopaminergic neurons in the substantia nigra. The most suggestive MRI feature of this disorder is absence of the normal "swallow tail" appearance of the substantia nigra on susceptibility weighted imaging. Typically, nigrosome-1, which contains the largest proportion of dopaminergic neurons affected in Parkinson's disease, demonstrates linear- or comma-shaped hyperintensity on susceptibility weighted imaging, but this is lost in Parkinson's disease. The symmetric middle cerebellar peduncle signal change is not characteristic of Parkinson's disease.

58.2 Correct: B. Expansion of a trinucleotide repeat in the untranslated region of the *FMR1* gene.

Both FXTAS and fragile X are associated with an excess of a normal CGC repeat sequence in the 5' untranslated region of the fragile-X mental-retardation 1 gene (*FMR1*). The *FMR1* premutation confers an increased risk of developing FXTAS; it is distinct from full mutation responsible for fragile X syndrome. Premutation alleles (55200 repeats) result in an excess of abnormal *FMR1* mRNA.

Other choices and discussion
C. Full mutation alleles (>200 repeats) trigger gene methylation and transcriptional silencing. Full mutations result in fragile-X syndrome, which is characterized by cognitive and behavioral problems, facial dysmorphism, and macro-orchidism.
A, E. Deletion of the *FMR* gene and deletion of the *FMR1* promoter have been implicated in fragile-X syndrome in several individuals, not FXTAS.
D. Missense mutation in the *FMR1* gene is incorrect.

58.3 Correct: C. X-linked dominant pattern.

FXTAS is inherited in an X-linked dominant pattern. The excess of abnormal *FMR1* mRNA in premutation alleles is thought to exert a toxic gain-of-function effect on various tissues including neurons and astrocytes.

Other choices and discussion
A, B, D, E. These answer choices are incorrect as the mode of inheritance for FXTAS is X-linked dominant.

References

Brunberg JA, Jacquemont S, Hagerman RJ, et al. Fragile-X Premutation Carriers: Characteristic MR Imaging Findings of Adult Male Patients with Progressive Cerebellar and Cognitive Dysfunction. *AJNR Am J Neuroradiol.* 2002;23(10):1757–1766.

Jacquemont S, Hagerman RJ, Hagerman PJ, et al. Fragile-X syndrome and fragile X-associated tremor/ataxia syndrome: two faces of FMR1. *Lancet Neurol.* 2007;6:45–55.

Case 59

Challenge

Please refer to the following images to answer the next three questions:

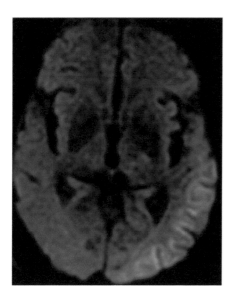 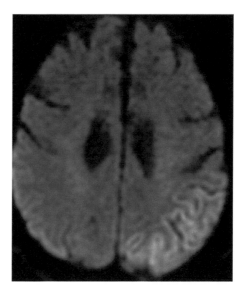

A 55-year-old male with prior history of basal ganglia infarction presents with acute onset global aphasia, left-sided weakness, and rightward eye deviation.

59.1 What is the **MOST** likely diagnosis?

A. Acute infarction.
B. Herpes simplex encephalitis.
C. Status epilepticus.
D. CreutzfeldtJakob disease (CJD).
E. Mitochondrial encephalomyopathy, lactic acidosis, and stroke-like episodes (MELAS).

59.2 What is the **MOST common** acute underlying etiology of status epilepticus in adults?

A. Stroke.
B. Metabolic abnormalities.
C. Hypoxia.
D. Systemic infection.
E. Trauma.

59.3 What is the overall mortality rate for status epilepticus in adults?

A. 10%.
B. 20%.
C. 30%.
D. 40%.
E. 50%.

Answers and Explanations

59.1   Correct: C. Status epilepticus.

Diffusion-weighted imaging (DWI) reveals mildly hyperintense signal in the left parietal, temporal, and occipital cortices. These findings, which are not constrained to a single vascular territory, are compatible with status epilepticus. In status epilepticus, restricted diffusion and T2/fluid-attenuated inversion recovery (FLAIR) hyperintensity can be seen in the ipsilateral (relative to the side of seizure onset) hippocampus, thalamus (particularly in the pulvinar nucleus), cerebral cortex and subcortical white matter, splenium of the corpus callosum, and contralateral cerebellum (due to corticocerebellar connections). Status epilepticus refers to prolonged or multiple seizures with incomplete return to baseline.

Other choices and discussion

A. In acute infarction, the area of restricted diffusion conforms to a vascular territory.

B. Typical MRI findings of herpes simplex encephalitis are bilateral and asymmetrical restricted diffusion and T2/FLAIR signal abnormality in the medial temporal and inferior frontal cortices. Hemorrhage and contrast enhancement may be present.

D. Hemorrhage and contrast enhancement may be present. CJD, the most common prion disease in humans, presents as a rapidly progressive dementia with an invariably fatal course within months to a year of diagnosis. Imaging findings include restricted diffusion involving the limbic system, neocortex, and deep gray matter. While there is some overlap with seizure-related cortical signal changes in status epilepticus, the clinical presentations differ.

E. MELAS is an inherited disorder, resulting from a mitochondrial DNA mutation that presents in childhood and adolescence with stroke-like episodes, seizures, and lactic acidosis. MRI shows cortical regions of restricted diffusion that may not necessarily conform to a vascular distribution and may disappear and reappear in different locations ("shifting spread").

59.2   Correct: A. Stroke.

Stroke is the most common acute underlying etiology of status epilepticus in adults.

Other choices and discussion

B–E. Metabolic abnormalities (**B**), hypoxia (**C**), systemic infection (**D**), and trauma (**E**) are other acute underlying etiologies of status epilepticus in adults but less common than stroke. Subtherapeutic levels of antiepileptic drugs in patients with chronic epilepsy, however, is the most common etiology of status epilepticus overall.

59.3   Correct: B. 20%.

The overall mortality rate for status epilepticus in adults is 20%.

Other choices and discussion

A, C, D, E. The other choices are incorrect. The underlying cause of status epilepticus is the most important determinant of mortality. Acute causes of status epilepticus are associated with higher mortality rates than chronic etiologies. The duration of seizure in status epilepticus also influences outcome, with higher morbidity and mortality associated with prolonged seizures (greater than 30 minutes).

References

Betjemann JP, Lowenstein DH. Status epilepticus in adults. *Lancet Neurol.* 2015;14:615–624.

Cartagena AM, Young GB, Lee DH. Reversible and irreversible cranial MRI findings associated with status epilepticus. *Epilepsy & Behavior.* 2014;33:24–30.

Milligan TA, Zamani A, Bromfeld E. Frequency and patterns of MRI abnormalities due to status epilepticus. *Seizure.* 2009;18:104–108.

Case 60

Challenge

Please refer to the following images to answer the next three questions:

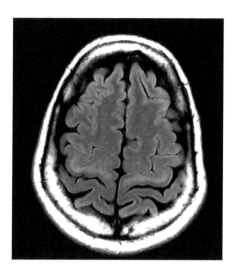 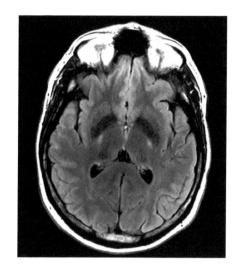

A 58-year-old male with no significant past medical history presents with slowly progressive upper and lower extremity fasciculations.

60.1   What is the **MOST** likely diawgnosis?

A. Amyotrophic lateral sclerosis (ALS).

B. Heroin-induced leukoencephalopathy.

C. Postanoxic leukoencephalopathy.

D. Methotrexate neurotoxicity.

E. Progressive multifocal leukoencephalopathy (PML).

60.2   What pattern of cerebral atrophy is seen in patients with ALS?

A. Parietal and temporal lobe atrophy.

B. Caudate and putamen atrophy.

C. Left anterior temporal lobe atrophy.

D. Frontal and temporal lobe atrophy.

E. Parietal and occipital lobe atrophy.

60.3   What condition can potentially mimic ALS both clinically and radiographically?

A. Multiple sclerosis (MS).

B. Cerebrovascular disease.

C. Celiac disease (CD).

D. Cervical spondylotic myelopathy.

E. Skull base lesions.

Answers and Explanations

60.1 Correct: A. Amyotrophic lateral sclerosis (ALS).

ALS is group of neurodegenerative disorders characterized by progressive loss of motor neurons, resulting in muscle weakness. The disease most frequently affects late middle-aged males and has a poor prognosis, with most patients surviving only 3 to 5 years following diagnosis. On MRI, signal abnormalities on T2-weighted, T2 fluid-attenuated inversion recovery (FLAIR), and proton density images are seen along the corticospinal tracts. The sensitivity of MRI for corticospinal tract (CST) signal changes varies but is only as high as 60%. Furthermore, signals along the CST have been described in normal controls, and in other conditions including Krabbe disease, X-linked CharcotMarie tooth neuropathies, adrenomyeloneuropathy, and celiac disease. As such, ALS remains a clinical diagnosis—the primary role of conventional neuroimaging is to exclude other causes that could explain the patient's presentation.

Other choices and discussion

B. Heroin-induced leukoencephalopathy is seen exclusively after heroin vapor inhalation ("chasing the dragon") and is characterized by white matter degeneration with preferential involvement of the posterior subcortical white matter, posterior limbs of the internal capsules, and cerebellar hemispheres.
C. Postanoxic leukoencephalopathy occurs in the days to weeks following an acute hypoxic event and is most frequently seen in association with carbon monoxide toxicity. Imaging demonstrates diffuse cerebral white matter injury with T2 FLAIR signal abnormality and diffusion restriction.
D. Methotrexate neurotoxicity can occur with high-dose intravenous or intrathecal methotrexate (MTX) administration and presents clinically with stroke-like symptoms. Imaging reveals asymmetric signal abnormalities in the frontoparietal white matter that are most obvious in the acute phase when there is diffusion restriction.
E. PML is an infectious demyelinating process, resulting from reactivation of the human polyomavirus JC, which occurs among immunocompromised patients. Imaging reveals geographic, multifocal, and asymmetric white matter lesions involving the subcortical-U fibers.

60.2 Correct: D. Frontal and temporal lobe atrophy.

While ALS is classically thought to be a pure motor disease, up to half of patients experience cognitive impairment, with 15% meeting criteria for frontotemporal dementia (FTD). Imaging studies have shown frontal and temporal cortical thinning in ALS patients, even among those without cognitive impairment. In patients with ALS-associated dementia, however, the degree of atrophy is more pronounced.

Other choices and discussion

A. Parietal and temporal lobe atrophy can be seen in Alzheimer's disease.
B. Caudate and putamen atrophy can be seen in Huntington's disease.
C. Unilateral left anterior temporal lobe atrophy can be seen in semantic variant primary progressive aphasia.
E. Parietal and occipital lobe atrophy can be seen in posterior cortical atrophy, often attributable to Alzheimer's disease, but they are also seen in association with dementia with Lewy bodies and corticobasal degeneration.

60.3 Correct: C. Celiac disease (CD).

CD, also known as celiac sprue, non-tropical sprue, and gluten-sensitive enteropathy, is an autoimmune inflammatory condition of the gastrointestinal tract. Some patients with CD also have neurological complications thought to be related to vitamin and mineral deficiency or, potentially, a neurotoxic autoimmune process. The most common CD-related neurologic symptoms are neuropathy and ataxia, but ALS and MS-like symptoms have also been reported. Imaging findings include T2/FLAIR signal abnormality along one or both corticospinal tracts, mimicking ALS, nonenhancing unilateral or bilateral T2/FLAIR periventricular white matter lesions, and occipital calcifications.

Other choices and discussion

A, B, D, E. Neuroimaging is performed in cases of clinically probable or possible ALS to exclude ALS-mimic syndromes, including Ms (**A**), cerebrovascular disease (**B**), cervical spondylotic myelopathy (**D**), and skull base lesions (**E**). These entities, however, have different imaging findings than ALS.

References

Agosta F, Chiò A, Cosottini M, et al. The Present and the Future of Neuroimaging in Amyotrophic Lateral Sclerosis. *AJNR Am J Neuroradiol.* 2010;31(10):1769–1777.

Brown KJ, Jewells V, Herfarth H, et al. White Matter Lesions Suggestive of Amyotrophic Lateral Sclerosis Attributed to Celiac Disease. *AJNR Am J Neuroradiol.* 2010;31(5):880–881.

Geibprasert S, Gallucci M, Krings T. Addictive Illegal Drugs: Structural Neuroimaging. *AJNR Am J Neuroradiol.* 2010;31(5):803–808.

Molloy S, Soh C, Williams TL. Reversible Delayed Posthypoxic Leukoencephalopathy. *AJNR Am J Neuroradiol.* 2006;27(8):1763–1765.

Crutch SJ, Lehmann M, Schott JM, et al. Posterior Cortical Atrophy. *Lancet Neurol.* 2012;11(2):170–178.

Case 61

Challenge

Please refer to the following images to answer the next three questions:

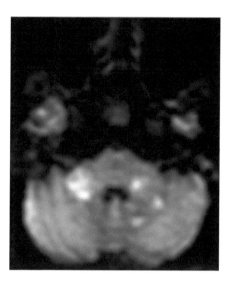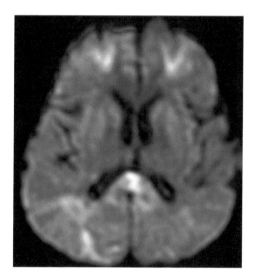

A 62-year-old male with progressive neurological decline over several months presents with paraplegia.

61.1 Which of the following is **NOT** in the differential diagnosis?

A. Primary angiitis of the central nervous system (PACNS).

B. Infectious vasculitis.

C. Creutzfeldt-Jakob disease (CJD).

D. Demyelinating disease.

E. Intravascular lymphoma (IVL).

61.2 What is the **MOST** common histology of intravascular lymphoma?

A. Myeloid precursor cell.

B. B-cell.

C. T-cell.

D. NK-cell.

E. Lymphoid precursor cell.

61.3 What is the prognosis of intravascular lymphoma?

A. Indolent course with greater than 10-year survival.

B. 5 to 10-year survival.

C. 1 to 5-year survival.

D. Several months.

E. Several weeks.

Answers and Explanations

61.1 Correct: C. Creutzfeldt-Jakob disease (CJD).

CJD is an important cause of rapidly progressive dementia. However, imaging findings in CJD include restricted diffusion and T2/fluid-attenuated inversion recovery (FLAIR) signal abnormality in the cortex, basal ganglia, and thalami.

Other choices and discussion

A. The typical parenchymal findings in PACNS are multiple subcortical infarctions, cortical infarctions, and infarcts in the deep gray matter, with less frequent involvement of the deep white matter and cerebellum. While this is not the best diagnosis for the given imaging findings, it can be included in the differential diagnosis.

B. Infectious vasculitis can occur in the setting of pyogenic, mycobacterial, fungal, and viral infections. In addition to the multifocal infarcts seen in end-organ injury related to vasculitis, there may also be evidence of infection on imaging, including leptomeningeal enhancement, focal parenchymal lesions (e.g., tuberculoma, cryptococcoma), or hydrocephalus.

D. Multifocal acute demyelinating lesions may be seen during a flare of multiple sclerosis (MS) or acute disseminated encephalomyelitis, or in the setting of progressive multifocal leukoencephalopathy (PML) for instance. Active lesions can restrict diffusion.

E. IVL is a rare malignancy characterized by aggregation and proliferation of tumor cells in small vessels. Within the CNS, IVL most commonly presents with multifocal infarct-like lesions with restricted diffusion throughout the cerebral white matter on MRI. IVL can also present with mass-like lesions, nonspecific T2 hyperintense lesions including involvement of the pons, linear enhancement along perivascular spaces, and meningeal enhancement. As IVL can clinically and radiographically mimic vasculitis and vascular dementia, biopsy is often required for definitive diagnosis. The patient above had a stereotactic biopsy revealing IVL.

61.2 Correct: B. B-cell.

The vast majority of IVLs are of B-cell origin (approximately 88%).

Other choices and discussion

C, D. Approximately 6% of IVLs are of T-cell (**C**) origin and approximately 2% of IVLs are of NK-cell (**D**) origin.

A, E. These choices are incorrect as the most common histology is of a B-cell origin.

61.3 Correct: D. Several months.

IVL has a poor prognosis; it is a rapidly progressive disease with a mortality rate greater than 80% and survival in the range of several months. This is, in part, due to the difficulty in diagnosis and suboptimal treatment, given the rarity of the disease. The other choices are incorrect.

Other choices and discussion

A–C, E. IVL does not follow an indolent course (**A**); rather it has a poor prognosis with an average survival rate of several months and not years (**B, C**) or weeks (**E**).

References

Fonken E, Lok E, Robison D, et al. The natural history of intravascular lymphoma. *Cancer Medicine.* 2014;3:1010–1024.

Pomper MG, Miller TJ, Stone JH, et al. CNS vasculitis in autoimmune disease: MR imaging findings and correlation with angiography. *AJNR Am J Neuroradiol.* 1999; 20: 75–85.

Ponzoni M, Ferreri AJ, Campo E, et al. Definition, diagnosis, and management of intravascular large B-cell lymphoma: proposals and perspectives from an international consensus meeting. *J Clin Oncol.* 2007;25:3168–3173.

Seby J, Hajj-Ali RA. CNS vasculitis. *Semin Neurol.* 2014;34:405–412.

Yamamoto A, Kikuchi Y, Homma K, et al. Characteristics of intravascular lymphoma on cerebral MR imaging. *AJNR Am J Neuroradiol.* 2012;33:292–296.

Case 62

Challenge

Please refer to the following images to answer the next three questions:

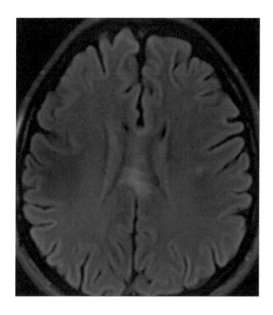 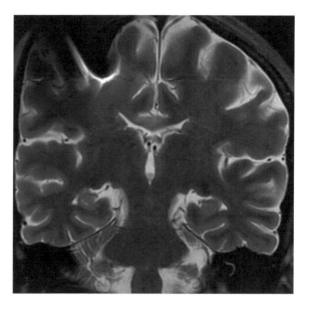

A 30-year-old female with history of hydrocephalus status post ventricular catheter placement.

62.1 What is the **MOST** likely etiology for the above findings?

A. Infiltration from "butterfly" neoplasm.

B. Destruction from progressive multifocal leukoencephalopathy (PML).

C. Chronic demyelination from osmotic demyelination syndrome.

D. Venous infarct.

E. Injury from long-standing compression due to hydrocephalus.

62.2 What is the **BEST** next step in management?

A. Do nothing.

B. Thrombolytic therapy.

C. Chemoradiation.

D. Follow-up MRI in 3 months.

E. Stereotactic biopsy.

62.3 With regard to patients with hydrocephalus, within how many hours does ventricular size return to normal following ventricular shunt placement?

A. 1 hour.

B. 12 hours.

C. 15 hours.

D. 24 hours.

E. 48 hours.

Answers and Explanations

62.1 Correct: E. Injury from long-standing compression due to hydrocephalus.

Abnormal signal changes within the corpus callosum in the setting of a patient with a ventriculoperitoneal shunt for significant hydrocephalus are thought to be due to long-standing compression of the fibers of the corpus callosum against the undersurface of the falx before ventricular decompression. This long-standing compression probably leads to venous or arterial ischemia which, in turn, leads to signal changes. In addition, this injury does not appear to produce or correlate with any clinical symptoms.

Other choices and discussion

A. The signal abnormality in the corpus callosum in this case does not appear mass-like, and there is no associated mass effect or perilesional edema to suggest infiltration from "butterfly" neoplasm. "Butterfly" brain tumors are those that extend across the corpus callosum to involve both cerebral hemispheres, often surrounding the ventricular system in a symmetrical pattern like the wings of a butterfly. These lesions, which are mass-like and frequently enhance, include lymphoma, high-grade astrocytoma or glioblastoma, and metastases.

B. Isolated corpus callosal involvement in an immunocompetent patient makes the diagnosis of PML very unlikely. Osmotic demyelination syndrome, formerly called central pontine and/or extrapontine myelinolysis, classically occurs after rapid correction of hyponatremia, although it can occur in normonatremic individuals. Common sites of extrapontine involvement include the cerebellum, thalami, basal ganglia, and cerebral white matter.

C. Isolated corpus callosum involvement from chronic osmotic demyelination is unlikely.

D. This lesion is not in a location typical of venous infarction.

62.2 Correct: A. Do nothing.

This is a do not touch lesion! Signal change of the corpus callosum from long-standing compression in a patient with hydrocephalus, who is currently shunted, does not appear to produce or correlate with any clinically recognizable symptoms. Therefore, there is nothing further to do with regard to management (treat the patient and not the imaging finding!). Notably, it is important to recognize this entity, so as to avoid misinterpreting the imaging findings as significant disease, which may lead to unnecessary intervention.

Other choices and discussion

B. Thrombolytic therapy is indicated in patients with acute stroke, which is not the case here.

C. Chemoradiation is not warranted as the corpus callosal signal is not due to an underlying tumor.

D. There is no need to do a follow-up MRI in this patient.

E. There is no need for a biopsy in this patient.

62.3 Correct: D. 24 hours.

Ventricular size typically returns to normal within 24 hours of ventricular shunt placement, although there may be a more gradual reduction in caliber depending on the chronicity and cause of hydrocephalus. If the lateral ventricles collapse too quickly, the brain may not be able to accommodate, leading to the formation of subdural hygromas or hematomas. Overdrainage is also common and can be suggested by slit-like ventricles on imaging. Other complications of shunting include meningeal fibrosis, ventriculitis, ventricular loculations, overdrainage, and shunt malfunctions (usually due to mechanical failures such as shunt occlusion, disconnections and breaks, and migration).

Other choices and discussion

A–C, E. The other answer choices are incorrect as ventricular size returns to normal within 24 hours of ventricular shunt placement as discussed above.

References

Destian S, Heier LA, Zimmerman RD, et al. Differentiation between meningeal fibrosis and chronic subdural hematoma after ventricular shunting: value of enhanced CT and MR scans. *AJNR Am J Neuroradiol.* 1989;10:1021–1026.

Goeser CD, McLeary MS, Young Lw. Diagnostic imaging of ventriculoperitoneal shunt malfunctions and complications. *Radiographics.* 1998;18:635–651.

Lane JI, Luetmer PH, Atkinson JL. Corpus callosal signal changes in patients with obstructive hydrocephalus after ventriculoperitoneal shunting. *AJNR Am J Neuroradiol.* 2001;22:158–162.

Middleton K, Esselman P, Lim PC. Terson syndrome: an underrecognized cause of reversible vision loss in patients with subarachnoid hemorrhage. *Am J Phys Med Rehabil.* 2012;91:271–274.

Wallace AN, McConathy J, Menias CO, et al. Imaging evaluation of CSF shunts. *AJR Am J Roentgenol.* 2014;202:38–53.

Case 63

Challenge

Please refer to the following images to answer the next three questions:

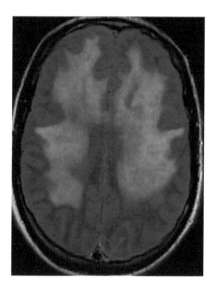 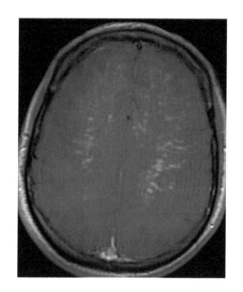

A 27-year-old with headaches and fever.

63.1 Which is the **LEAST** likely diagnosis?

A. Lymphoma.
B. Vasculitis.
C. Progressive multifocal leukoencephalopathy (PML).
D. HIV encephalopathy.
E. Acute disseminated encephalomyelitis (ADEM).

63.2 Which of the following statements regarding intravascular lymphoma is **TRUE**?

A. Commonly seen in young patients.
B. Often mimics vasculitis on imaging.
C. Stroke-like symptoms are the most common clinical presentation.
D. Central nervous system (CNS) involvement is rare.
E. Generally has a good prognosis.

63.3 Which of the following statements regarding granulomatosis with polyangitis (GPA) is **TRUE**?

A. Brain biopsy may be required to confirm diagnosis.
B. 90% of cases are perinuclear anti-neutrophil cytoplasmic antibodies (P-ANCA) positive.
C. CNS involvement is common.
D. Treated with radiation therapy.
E. Large vessel vasculitis.

Answers and Explanations

63.1 Correct: D. HIV encephalopathy.

HIV encephalopathy typically presents with nonenhancing confluent white matter T2 hyperintensities and volume loss which may be advanced for age–findings that can correlate clinically with early onset dementia. In the above case, the presence of enhancement makes HIV encephalopathy the LEAST likely diagnosis in this scenario.

Other choices and discussion

A, B. T2 fluid-attenuated inversion recovery (FLAIR) image demonstrates confluent white matter hyperintensity with involvement of both the subcortical and deep white matter. Postcontrast T1 image demonstrates multiple linear enhancing foci within the regions of white matter signal abnormality. These findings can be seen with both angiocentric lymphoma and vasculitis.

The above case represents biopsy-proven granulomatosis with polyangiitis (GPA). The imaging findings of vasculitis were better appreciated on magnetic resonance (MR) angiogram and conventional angiography (images not provided).

C. PML represents an opportunistic infection by John Cunningham (JC) virus in immunocompromised patients, manifesting as confluent white matter T2 hyperintensities with characteristic involvement of the subcortical U-fibers, generally without enhancement. However, enhancement can be seen with immune reconstitution (IRIS immune reconstitution inflammatory syndrome) or chronic PML infection. Hence, PML is not the LEAST likely diagnosis.

E. Acute demyelinating encephalomyelitis represents acute demyelination days to weeks following infection or vaccination, with punctate or ring-like enhancing lesions and surrounding white matter T2 hyperintensity within the deep white matter as well as the basal ganglia. Cord lesions can also be seen.

63.2 Correct: B. Often mimics vasculitis on imaging.

Intravascular (angiocentric) lymphoma is a rare and aggressive non-Hodgkin's lymphoma that often mimics vasculitis and vascular dementia on imaging. Imaging findings can be nonspecific and include multifocal T2 FLAIR white matter hyperintensities, diffusion restriction, and multifocal perivascular hemorrhage, with associated linear or mass-like enhancement. The underlying pathology is related to arterial and venous occlusion from angiotropic growth of malignant lymphoid cells. Diagnosis can be made from skin or brain biopsy. Treatment includes chemotherapy and steroids, similar to primary and secondary CNS lymphoma.

Other choices and discussion

A. Intravascular lymphoma usually presents in the 5th to 7th decades of life.

C. Dementia is the most common clinical manifestation, although patients can also present with stroke-like or nonspecific symptoms.

D. Intravascular lymphoma commonly involves the brain (75% of cases involve the CNS) and skin.

E. Intravascular lymphoma is a rapidly progressive disease with a high-mortality rate.

63.3 Correct: A. Brain biopsy may be required to confirm diagnosis.

GPA, formerly known as Wegener granulomatosis, is a cytoplasmic antineutrophil cytoplasmic autoantibody (C-ANCA)-positive small-medium vessel autoimmune vasculitis commonly involving the lungs and kidneys. CNS manifestations are rare and seen in approximately 5% of the patients. CNS manifestations include small vessel vasculitis (presenting with perivascular enhancement and T2 FLAIR white matter hyperintensities) and granulomas involving the parenchyma and meninges. A brain biopsy is often necessary to confirm the diagnosis, given the nonspecific imaging findings. Treatment includes immunosuppressive medications such as steroids, methotrexate, and cyclophosphamide.

Other choices and discussion

B. GPA, formerly known as Wegener granulomatosis, is a cytoplasmic antineutrophil cytoplasmic autoantibody (C-ANCA)-positive small-to-medium vessel autoimmune vasculitis commonly involving the lungs and kidneys.

C. CNS manifestations are rare and seen in approximately 5% of the patients. CNS manifestations include small-to-medium vessel vasculitis (presenting with perivascular enhancement and T2 FLAIR white matter hyperintensities) and granulomas involving the parenchyma and meninges.

D. Treatment includes immunosuppressive medications such as steroids, methotrexate, and cyclophosphamide.

E. GPA is a small-to-medium vessel vasculitis.

References

De Luna G, Terrier B, Kaminsky P, et al. Central nervous system involvement of granulomatosis with polyangiitis: clinical-radiological presentation distinguishes different outcomes. *Rheumatology (Oxford)*. 2015;54(3):424–432.

Mahan M, Karl M, Gordon S. Neuroimaging of viral infections of the central nervous **system**. *Handb Clin Neurol*. 2014;123:149–173.

Shimada K, Murase T, Matsue K, et al. Central nervous system involvement in intravascular large B-cell lymphoma: a retrospective analysis of 109 patients. *Cancer Sci*. 2010;101(6):1480-1486.

Yamamoto A, Kikuchi Y, Homma K, et al. Characteristics of intravascular large B-cell lymphoma on cerebral MR imaging. *AJNR Am J Neuroradiol*. 2012;33(2):292-296.

Case 64

Challenge

Please refer to the following images to answer the next three questions:

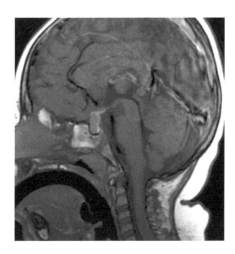 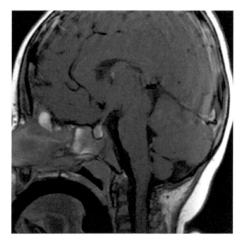

An 18-month-old with hypotonia, jaundice, decreased activity, and failure to thrive. The first image was obtained at time of presentation and the second image was obtained 3 months after intervention.

64.1 What is considered the normal upper limit of the height of pituitary gland in an infant?

A. 4 mm.

B. 6 mm.

C. 8 mm.

D. 10 mm.

E. 12 mm.

64.2 What was the **MOST** likely treatment in this case given the patient's age, clinical presentation, and imaging findings?

A. Surgical removal of tumor.

B. Cabergoline.

C. Estrogen hormone replacement.

D. Radiation therapy.

E. Thyroid hormone replacement.

64.3 Which of the following conditions can cause pituitary hyperplasia?

A. Addison disease.

B. Hyperthyroidism.

C. Hyperparathyroidism.

D. Hypoparathyroidism.

E. Menopause

Answers and Explanations

64.1 Correct: B. 6 mm.

6 mm is considered the upper limit of a normal pituitary height in infants and children.

Other choices and discussion

A, C–E. The other answer choices are incorrect. 8 mm (C) is considered the upper limit of normal in postmenopausal women and males, and 10 mm (D) is the upper limit in menstruating females, related to physiologically elevated estrogen levels. The pituitary gland can physiologically enlarge up to 12 mm (E), with a convex upper margin in pregnant and lactating females due to complex hormonal changes in these states. 4 mm (A) is not a relevant number in this setting. Height of the pituitary gland greater than that expected for a specific age and/or sex should raise a concern for an underlying lesion.

64.2 Correct: E. Thyroid hormone replacement.

The first (postcontrast T1-weighted) image demonstrates a homogenously enlarged anterior pituitary with suprasellar extension, lifting of the pituitary stalk and hypothalamic tuber cinereum, and a normal posterior pituitary "bright spot." There is mass effect on the optic pathway which is not well-appreciated on the provided image. Based on the patient's clinical presentation and laboratory data, the imaging findings are most concerning for pituitary hyperplasia related to hypothyroidism. The patient was treated with thyroid hormone replacement, which led to clinical improvement as well as a significant decrease in size of the pituitary gland on the 3-month follow-up scan (second image).

Other choices and discussion

A–D. Answer choices are incorrect. Pituitary adenomas are uncommon in the pediatric population and, therefore,

the clinical history does not raise the concern for a prolactinoma, which would be treated with cabergoline (B). No surgical changes (A) are seen on the second image to suggest trans-sphenoidal resection of a lesion. Radiation therapy (D) or estrogen replacement (C) are not relevant in this clinical setting.

64.3 Correct: A. Addison disease.

Pituitary hyperplasia is seen in infants and children in the setting of end-organ failure. Answer choice (A) is correct since adrenal insufficiency, similar to hypothyroidism, can lead to pituitary hyperplasia from excessive and uninhibited production of corticotropin-releasing hormone from the hypothalamus.

Other choices and discussion

B–E. The other answer choices are incorrect. Hyperthyroidism (B) would lead to suppression of the pituitary gland. Parathyroid hormone (CD) axis does not involve the pituitary gland. Decreased production of estrogen leads to menopause (E), which would not lead to pituitary hyperplasia.

References

Hutchins WW, Crues JV, Miya P, et al. MR demonstration of pituitary hyperplasia and regression after therapy for hypothyroidism. *AJNR Am J Neuroradiol.* 1990;11(20):410.

Siddiqi AI, Grieve J, Miszkiel K, et al. Tablets or scalpel: Pituitary hyperplasia due to primary hypothyroidism. *Radiology Case Reports.* 2015;2:1099.

Tsunoda A, Okuda O, Sato K. MR height of the pituitary gland as a function of age and sex: especially physiological hypertrophy in adolescence and in climacterium. *AJNR Am J Neuroradiol.* 1997;18(3):551-554.

Case 65

Challenge

Please refer to the following images to answer the next three questions:

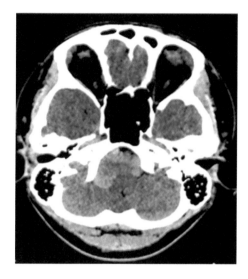

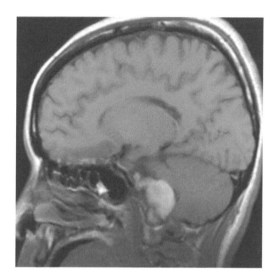

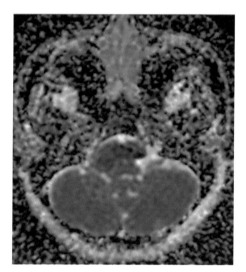

A 30-year-old man with headaches.

65.1 The images demonstrate which of the following?

A. Intra-axial mass.

B. Diffusion restriction.

C. Enhancement.

D. Osseous lesion.

E. Calcification.

65.2 What are the two **MOST** likely differential considerations based on the imaging characteristics and location of this lesion?

A. Arachnoid cyst and dermoid cyst.

B. Epidermoid cyst and colloid cyst.

C. Ecchordosis physaliphora and neurenteric cyst.

D. Epidermoid cyst and neurenteric cyst.

E. Chordoma and arachnoid cyst.

65.3 Which of the cyst contents can explain both the T1 hyperintensity and CT hyperdensity in an epidermoid?

A. Triglycerides.

B. Keratin filaments.

C. Protein.

D. Fatty acids.

E. CSF.

Answers and Explanations

65.1 Correct: B. Diffusion restriction.

The apparent diffusion coefficient (ADC) map demonstrates mild diffusion restriction within an extra-axial lesion within the retroclival region.

Other choices and discussion

A. The lesion is extra-axial, not intra-axial, in location.

C. The second image is a precontrast T1 image, given the absence of contrast enhancement of the brain parenchyma, vessels, as well as the nasal mucosa, which shows intrinsic T1 hyperintensity within the lesion. No postcontrast imaging is provided.

D. No osseous involvement is demonstrated.

E. Although the lesion is hyperdense on CT, no definite internal calcifications are seen.

65.2 Correct: D. Epidermoid cyst and neurenteric cyst.

The images demonstrate a lobulated, hyperdense, midline extra-axial mass within the prepontine and premedullary cisterns, demonstrating mild diffusion restriction and T1 shortening. The primary differential consideration would be a neurenteric cyst based on the midline retroclival location, CT hyperdensity, and T1 shortening. Neurenteric cysts can rarely demonstrate mild diffusion restriction. However, these imaging findings can also be explained by an atypical, "white" epidermoid cyst, which gets its name from the underlying T1 shortening. "White" epidermoids can also be hyperdense on CT, in addition to demonstrating diffusion restriction, which is the hallmark finding of epidermoid cysts. This lesion proved to be an epidermoid on biopsy.

Other choices and discussion

A–C, E. Other answer choices are incorrect. Arachnoid cysts should follow cerebrospinal fluid (CSF) intensity on all sequences, although they can be hyperdense on CT and T1 hyperintense if there is underlying hemorrhage. However, arachnoid cysts should not demonstrate diffusion restriction. Dermoid cysts are fat-containing and hence can be T1 hyperintense on magnetic resonance imaging (MRI). However, no fat density is present on the CT image, which excludes this diagnosis. Colloid cysts can be hyperdense on CT and T1 hyperintense. However, greater than 99% of colloid cysts are seen along the foramen of Monro. Extraventricular colloid cysts are extremely rare. The retroclival location is ideal for ecchordosis physaliphora which is a notochord remnant. However, no dorsal clival osseous stalk or defect is seen to support this diagnosis. In addition, ecchordosis generally follows CSF intensity on all sequences, similar to an arachnoid cyst. Chordomas are locally aggressive tumors originating from notochordal remnants that clinically present with skull base invasion. The images demonstrate a benign-appearing lesion that does not invade the clivus.

65.3 Correct: C. Protein.

Atypical, "white" epidermoids get their name from the intrinsic T1 hyperintensity, which can either be related to proteinaceous contents or triglycerides and fatty acids. Noncontrast CT can differentiate between these two types of "white" epidermoids. Proteinaceous contents within an epidermoid cyst are hyperdense on CT, hyperintense or hypointense on T2, and T1 hyperintense.

Other choices and discussion

A, D. Triglycerides and fatty acids can be T1 hyperintense, with a drop in signal on fat-suppressed sequences, but will be hypodense on CT.

B. Keratin filaments are responsible for the hallmark finding of diffusion restriction within epidermoids and contribute to T1 hypointense signal.

E. CSF is hypodense on CT and T1 hypointense.

References

Ben Hamouda M, Drissi C, Sebai R, et al. Atypical CT and MRI aspects of an epidermoid cyst. *J Neuroradiol.* 2007;34(2):129–132.

Chen CY, Wong JS, Hsieh SC, et al. Intracranial epidermoid cyst with hemorrhage: MR imaging findings. *AJNR Am J Neuroradiol.* 2006;27(2):427–429.

Medhi G, Saini J, Pandey P, et al. T1 hyperintense prepontine mass with restricted diffusion: a white epidermoid or a neuroenteric cyst? *J Neuroimaging.* 2015;25(5):841–843.

Preece MT, Osborn AG, Chin SS, et al. Intracranial neurenteric cysts: imaging and pathology spectrum. *AJNR Am J Neuroradiol.* 2006;27(6):1211–1216.

Case 66

Challenge

Please refer to the following images to answer the next three questions:

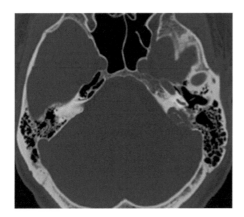
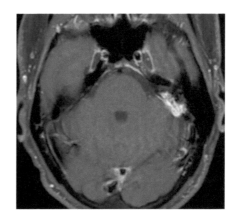

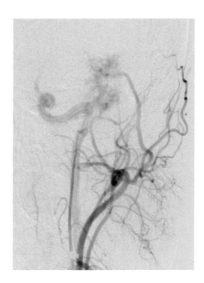

A 46-year-old male presents with pulsatile tinnitus and vertigo.

66.1 What is the **MOST** likely diagnosis?

A. Vestibular schwannoma.

B. Glomus jugulare paraganglioma.

C. Endolymphatic sac tumor.

D. Meningioma.

E. Glomus tympanicum paraganglioma.

66.2 The third image demonstrates a digital subtraction angiogram of which vessel?

A. Right vertebral artery.

B. Left external carotid artery.

C. Right internal carotid artery.

D. Left internal carotid artery.

E. Left vertebral artery.

66.3 Which of the following statements regarding Von Hippel Lindau (VHL) syndrome is **TRUE**?

A. Endolymphatic sac tumors are seen in 30% of VHL patients.

B. Retinal detachment is uncommon at a young age.

C. Hemangioblastomas arise from deep white matter.

D. Autosomal recessive inheritance.

E. Enlargement of the cystic component of a hemangioblastoma is an indicator of tumor growth.

Answers and Explanations

66.1   Correct: C. Endolymphatic sac tumor.

The CT image shows a locally destructive lytic lesion involving the posterior aspect of the left petrous temporal bone. The lesion demonstrates avid enhancement on postcontrast T1-weighted imaging. The digital subtraction angiogram in the third image shows that the tumor is hypervascular.

Other choices and discussion

E, B. Glomus tympanicum (**E**) and glomus jugulare (**B**) paragangliomas are also highly vascular tumors; however, the key in differentiating between these three lesions is the anatomic location. The posterior aspect of the petrous temporal bone, posteromedial to the cochlea in the region of the vestibular aqueduct, is a characteristic location for an endolymphatic sac tumor. Glomus tympanicum tumors arise from the Jacobson nerve at the cochlear promontory and hence are seen lateral to the cochlea, possibly involving the middle ear cavity. Glomus jugulare tumors are centered at the jugular bulb rather than the posterior petrous bone.

D. The imaging characteristics are not typical for a meningioma, which is typically associated with bony hyperostosis (not seen on the CT image).

A. This is an incorrect option because no enhancing nodule is seen within the left internal auditory canal, which is located anterior to the lesion on the postcontrast T1-weighted image.

66.2   Correct: B. Left external carotid artery.

The anterior-posterior digital subtraction angiogram of the left external carotid artery demonstrates supply to the hypervascular tumor from its branches.

Other choices and discussion

A, C. This is an anterior-posterior or frontal view of the digital subtraction angiogram. As such, the selected vessel is on the radiographic left (and not right) side of the patient.

D. Although there is some contrast opacification of the left internal carotid artery due to reflux of contrast dye, there is more robust opacification of the left external carotid artery from selective injection of this vessel.

E. The digital subtraction angiogram does not show opacification of the left vertebral artery and posterior circulation.

66.3   Correct: E. Enlargement of the cystic component of a hemangioblastoma is an indicator of tumor growth.

Hemangioblastomas can demonstrate periods of progressive enlargement with intervening periods of arrested growth. On average, new lesions develop every 2 years. Increased size of the cystic component is often accompanied by increased size of the solid component; it is a marker for growth on follow-up imaging. Hemangioblastomas arise from the pial surface and hence tend to present as superficial lesions.

Other choices and discussion

D. VHL is an autosomal dominant familial syndrome characterized by benign cysts within visceral organs, vascular tumors including central nervous system hemangioblastomas, and carcinomas. Hemangioblastomas can demonstrate periods of progressive enlargement with intervening periods of arrested growth. On average, new lesions develop every 2 years. Increased size of the cystic component is often accompanied by increased size of the solid component; it is a marker for growth on follow-up imaging. Hemangioblastomas arise from the pial surface and hence tend to present as superficial lesions.

C. Lesions located solely within deep white matter should raise the concern for other primary central nervous system (CNS) neoplasms.

A. The prevalence of endolymphatic sac tumors is only 4% in patients with VHL.

B. Visual symptoms related to retinal hemorrhage and detachment from underlying retinal angiomas are common and often the earliest manifestation of VHL.

References

Leung RS, Biswas SV, Duncan M, et al. Imaging features of von Hippel-Lindau disease. *Radiographics*. 2008;28(1): 65–79.

Lonser RR, Kim HJ, Butman JA, et al. Tumors of the endolymphatic sac in von Hippel-Lindau disease. *N. Engl. J. Med.* 2004;350(24): 2481–2486.

Case 67

Challenge

Please refer to the following images to answer the next three questions:

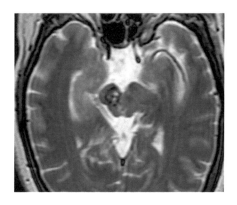 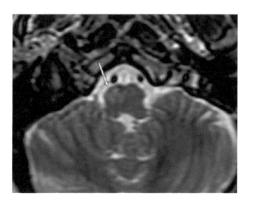

A 42-year-old male with headaches.

67.1 What is the **MOST** likely diagnosis on the first image?

A. Pilocytic astrocytoma.

B. Acute parenchymal hemorrhage.

C. Parasitic cyst.

D. Cavernous malformation.

E. Hypertensive microangiopathy.

67.2 Which structure is the arrow pointing to on the second image?

A. Inferior cerebellar peduncle.

B. Inferior olivary nucleus.

C. Superior cerebellar peduncle.

D. Cerebral peduncle.

E. Red nucleus.

67.3 What is the classic clinical presentation in a patient with hypertrophic olivary degeneration?

A. Lower extremity weakness.

B. Psychosis.

C. Generalized tremor.

D. Locked-in syndrome.

E. Palatal myoclonus.

Answers and Explanations

67.1 Correct: D. Cavernous malformation.

Axial T2 image demonstrates a "bubbly" T2 hyperintense lesion surrounded by a rim of T2 hypointense signal in the right cerebral peduncle. The rim of T2 hypointensity is related to chronic hemosiderin staining due to multiple episodes of repeated localized hemorrhage. Imaging findings are characteristic of a cavernous malformation.

Other choices and discussion

A. A pilocytic astrocytoma is typically seen in the pediatric population and presents as a cyst with an enhancing mural nodule.
B. Acute parenchymal hemorrhage is T1 isohypointense and T2 hypointense; however, the T2 hypointensity is not organized as in a cavernous malformation.
C. Although calcified neurocysticercal cysts (nodular calcified stage) can be T2 hypointense, they usually present as a focal calcified nodule without internal T2 hyperintense foci.
E. Hypertensive microangiopathy commonly involves the brainstem and can be associated with chronic microhemorrhage and hemosiderin deposition but does not usually present as a "bubbly" lesion containing T2 hyperintense foci.

67.2 Correct: B. Inferior olivary nucleus.

The arrow in the second image points to the inferior olivary nucleus.

Other choices and discussion

A, C–E. The other answer choices are incorrect. There is slight enlargement and T2 hyperintensity of the right inferior olivary nucleus, which represents hypertrophic degeneration. Hypertrophic olivary degeneration (HOD) is a unique form of trans-synaptic neuronal degeneration caused by lesions within the triangle of Guillain–Molaret, which is defined by the olivary nucleus, ipsilateral red nucleus, and contralateral dentate nucleus. The cavernous malformation in the first image likely involves the right red nucleus within the midbrain and disrupts the central tegmental tract that connects the red nucleus to the ipsilateral olivary nucleus, causing neuronal degeneration. The olivary nucleus hypertrophies can remain in this state for years and may eventually atrophy. Contralateral HOD can be seen if the primary lesion is within the cerebellum. Bilateral lesions can be seen if there is disruption of the central tegmental tract as well as the superior cerebellar peduncle (which contains the dentorubral tract connecting the dentate nucleus to the contralateral red nucleus). HOD can also manifest after removal of a brainstem or cerebellar cavernous malformation. It is important to correctly identify this lesion and recommend follow-up instead of incorrectly labeling it an infarct, neoplasm, or demyelinating plaque.

67.3 Correct: E. Palatal myoclonus.

Palatal myoclonus is a classic clinical finding in a patient with HOD. Virtually all patients with palatal myoclonus will have HOD on imaging, whereas not all patients with HOD present with this symptom. Palatal tremors typically develop about 10 months after hypertrophic degeneration of the inferior olivary nucleus. Patients present with rhythmic involuntary movements of the soft palate, uvula, pharynx and larynx, and clinical symptoms rarely improve despite temporal evolution of HOD.

Other choices and discussion

A–D. Other answer choices are not classic clinical manifestations of HOD.

References

Goyal M, Versnick E, Tuite P, et al. Hypertrophic olivary degeneration: metaanalysis of the temporal evolution of MR findings. *AJNR Am J Neuroradiol.* 2000;21(6):1073-1077.

Hornyak M, Osborn AG, Couldwell WT. Hypertrophic olivary degeneration after surgical removal of cavernous malformations of the brain stem: report of four cases and review of the literature. *Acta Neurochir (Wien).* 2008;150(2):149–156; discussion 156.

Mokin M, Agazzi S, Dawson L, et al. Neuroimaging of cavernous malformations. *Curr Pain Headache Rep.* 2017;21(12):47.

Palacios E, Wasilewska E, Alvernia JE, et al. Palatal myoclonus secondary to hypertrophic olivary degeneration. *Ear Nose Throat J.* 2009;88(7):989-991.

Case 68

Challenge

Please refer to the following images to answer the next three questions:

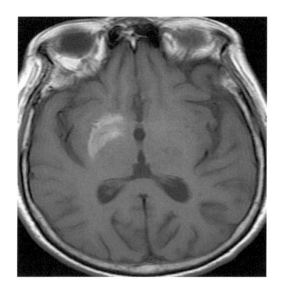 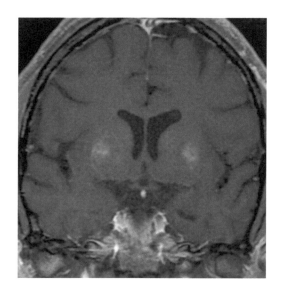

The first and second images are from two different patients with uncontrolled type II diabetes, who present with altered mental status, jerky involuntary movements, and blood glucose between 360 and 400 mg/dL.

68.1 Which of the following conditions does **NOT** present with T1 hyperintense basal ganglia?

A. Hyperalimentation.

B. Multiple postcontrast MRI examinations.

C. Hepatic encephalopathy.

D. Acute renal failure.

E. Neurofibromatosis type I.

68.2 What is the **MOST** likely diagnosis based on the provided clinical scenario?

A. Diabetic nephropathy.

B. Carbon monoxide poisoning.

C. Diabetic striatopathy.

D. Diabetic ketoacidosis.

E. Cirrhosis.

68.3 Which of the following statements regarding non-ketotic hyperglycemic hemichorea is **TRUE**?

A. Lesions can demonstrate restricted diffusion.

B. Imaging findings are almost always bilateral.

C. Symptoms do not resolve despite correction of hyperglycemia.

D. Presents with sensory symptoms.

E. Most consistent imaging finding is T1 hyperintensity of the thalamus.

Answers and Explanations

68.1 Correct: D. Acute renal failure.

Basal ganglia signal abnormalities are not typically seen in patients with acute renal failure.

Other choices and discussion

A–C. Patients afflicted with chronic renal failure and on hemodialysis can present with T1 hyperintense basal ganglia related to deposition of manganese, which is also seen in patients with hepatic encephalopathy (**C**) and those receiving hyperalimentation therapy (**A**). Patients undergoing multiple contrast-enhanced MRI examinations (**B**) show T1 hyperintensity within the basal ganglia and dentate nucleus, presumably related to deposition of gadolinium.

E. Symmetric T1 hyperintense basal ganglia lesions can be seen in patients with neurofibromatosis type I.

68.2 Correct: C. Diabetic striatopathy.

The first image is an axial noncontrast T1-weighted image which demonstrates hyperintensity within the right lentiform nucleus. The second image is an axial postcontrast T1-weighted image from a different patient which demonstrates increased signal within both putamina, which was intrinsically T1 hyperintense when correlated with the noncontrast T1 (not provided). The most likely diagnosis in both cases is diabetic striatopathy, which is also known as non-ketotic hyperglycemic hemichorea. Patients present with rapid onset of unilateral or bilateral chorea during an episode of nonketotic hyperglycemia. T1 hyperintensity of the putamen and caudate tends to be the most common imaging finding, although the underlying etiology is poorly understood. When the imaging finding is unilateral, symptoms are seen on the contralateral side. Symptoms are seen on the contralateral side in unilateral lesions. Upon correction of hyperglycemia, symptoms typically resolve earlier than the imaging findings.

Other choices and discussion

A. Patients with diabetic nephropathy can present with basal ganglia T1 signal abnormalities related to chronic renal failure and longstanding hemodialysis; however, this is not the most likely diagnosis based on the provided clinical scenario.

D. Diabetic ketoacidosis can manifest with cerebral edema and infarction in the pediatric population.

B, E. Answer choices can cause basal ganglia signal abnormalities but do not fit the clinical scenario and are incorrect.

68.3 Correct: A. Lesions can demonstrate restricted diffusion.

Although T1 hyperintensity within the putamen and caudate is the most common imaging finding, mild restricted diffusion has been reported.

Other choices and discussion

E. T1 hyperintensity of the thalamus has not been reported.

C. Symptoms generally resolve upon correction of hyperglycemia.

B. Imaging findings can be either unilateral or bilateral.

D. Patients can have altered mental status but do not present with sensory symptoms.

References

Hansford BG, Albert D, Yang E. Classic neuroimaging findings of nonketotic hyperglycemia on computed tomography and magnetic resonance imaging with absence of typical movement disorder symptoms (hemichorea-hemiballism). *J Radiol Case Rep.* 2013;7(8):1–9.

Hegde AN, Mohan S, Lath N, et al. Differential diagnosis for bilateral abnormalities of the basal ganglia and thalamus. *Radiographics.* 2011;31(1):5–30.

Wintermark M, Fischbein NJ, Mukherjee P, et al. Unilateral putaminal CT, MR, and diffusion abnormalities secondary to nonketotic hyperglycemia in the setting of acute neurologic symptoms mimicking stroke. *AJNR Am J Neuroradiol.* 2004;25(6):975–976.

Case 69

Challenge

Please refer to the following images to answer the next three questions:

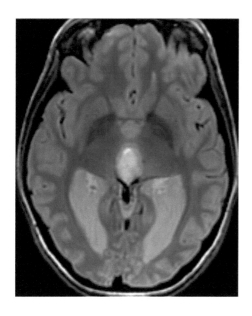

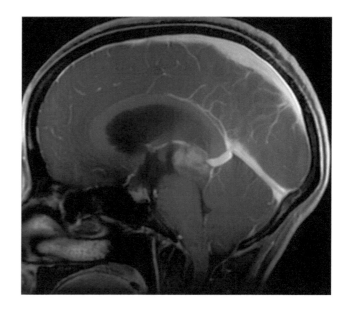

A 33-year-old female presents with Parinaud syndrome.

69.1 What is the **MOST** likely diagnosis?

A. Pineal parenchymal tumor of intermediate differentiation.
B. Pineoblastoma.
C. Germinoma.
D. Pineocytoma.
E. Normal pineal gland.

69.2 Which of the following borders the pineal gland?

A. Tegmentum.
B. Ambient cistern.
C. Midbrain.
D. Internal cerebral veins.
E. Fourth ventricle.

69.3 Which of the following is **TRUE** regarding the imaging appearance of this entity?

A. Invasion of adjacent structures is common.
B. Pineal calcifications appear "exploded."
C. Avid homogeneous enhancement is present.
D. Size criterion is >1.5 cm.
E. Magnetic resonance spectroscopy shows increased N-acetyl aspartate (NAA).

Answers and Explanations

69.1 Correct: A. Pineal parenchymal tumor of intermediate differentiation.

On the axial T2-weighted and sagittal postcontrast T1-weighted images, there is a heterogeneously enhancing pineal region mass, causing mass effect on the cerebral aqueduct and moderate obstructive hydrocephalus.

Other choices and discussion

D, B. When encountering an aggressive pineal mass in an adult, the diagnosis of pineal parenchymal tumor of intermediate differentiation (PPTID) is most likely. This tumor type is intermediate between pineocytoma (**D**), which is a slow-growing tumor with a good prognosis, and pineoblastoma (**B**), which is an aggressive-appearing tumor that occurs predominantly in children.
C. Germinomas are typically seen in adolescent male patients, rendering this diagnosis unlikely in a 33-year-old female.
E. The pineal gland in this case is not normal by size or enhancement pattern.

69.2 Correct: D. Internal cerebral veins.

The internal cerebral veins run along the superior aspect of the pineal gland.

Other choices and discussion

E. The third, not the fourth, ventricle is immediately anterior to the pineal gland; third ventricular masses displace the pineal gland posteriorly.
B. The quadrigeminal cistern, not the ambient cistern, is located posterior to the pineal gland.
A. The tegmentum is located ventral to the cerebral aqueduct and does not directly border the pineal gland. In contrast, the tectum is dorsal to the cerebral aqueduct and lies below the pineal gland; therefore, tectal lesions displace the pineal gland superiorly.
C. The midbrain is anterior to but does not immediately border the pineal gland.

69.3 Correct: A. Invasion of adjacent structures is common.

Invasion of adjacent structures, such as the ventricles, thalami, and tectum, is common.

Other choices and discussion

B. The calcifications appear "engulfed" in pineal parenchymal tumors of intermediate differentiation and are best demonstrated on CT. In contrast, the calcifications appear "exploded" in pineoblastomas.
C. In contrast, the calcifications appear "exploded" in pineoblastomas. There is strong enhancement in PPTID, but the enhancement is heterogeneous and not homogeneous.
D. PPTID has no size criterion, and tumors can range from subcentimeter to greater than 6 cm.
E. The NAA peak is decreased on MR spectroscopy, which is true for most intracranial tumors.

References

Komakula S, Warmuth-Metz M, Hildenbrand P, et al. Pineal parenchymal tumor of intermediate differentiation: imaging spectrum of an unusual tumor in 11 cases. *Neuroradiology*. 2011;53:577.

Osborn AG. Pineal and Germ Cell Tumors. In: Osborn AG, Hedlund GL, editors. Osborn's Brain: Imaging, Pathology, and Anatomy. 2nd ed. Philadelphia: Elsevier; 2018: 608–618.

Case 70

Challenge

Please refer to the following images to answer the next three questions:

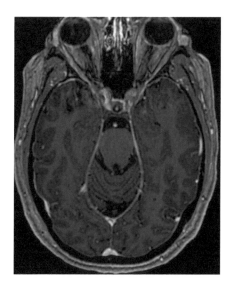

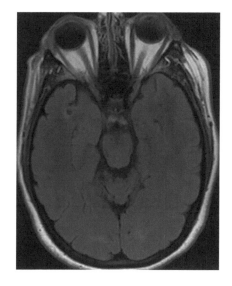

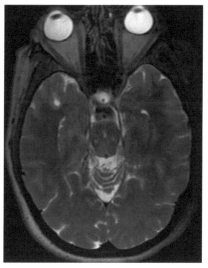

A 35-year-old female with memory loss.

70.1 What is the **MOST** likely diagnosis?

A. Glioependymal cyst.
B. Neuroglial cyst.
C. Anterior temporal lobe perivascular space.
D. Arachnoid cyst.
E. Astrocytoma.

70.2 Which of the following describes the lesion's imaging appearance?

A. Lack of perilesional T2/FLAIR hyperintensity.

B. Gradual increase in size over time.
C. Homogeneous enhancement.
D. Adjacent to a branch of the middle cerebral artery.
E. Restricted diffusion.

70.3 What is the **MOST** common location for an enlarged perivascular space?

A. Subcortical white matter.
B. Anterior temporal lobe.
C. Dentate nucleus of the cerebellum.
D. Midbrain.
E. Inferior third of the basal ganglia.

Answers and Explanations

70.1 Correct: C. Anterior temporal lobe perivascular space.

On the axial T1-weighted postcontrast and fluid-attenuated inversion recovery (FLAIR) images, there is a round cerebrospinal fluid (CSF)-intensity lesion in the anterior superior temporal gyrus, with mild surrounding perilesional FLAIR signal. This appearance and location is classic for the recently recognized entity of the anterior temporal lobe perivascular space.

Other choices and discussion
A. The glioependymal cyst appears similar but has a predilection for juxtraventricular locations.
B. The neuroglial cyst also appears similar but has a predilection for the frontal lobe.
D. An arachnoid cyst is not expected to have surrounding FLAIR signal.
E. Astrocytoma is possible, although less likely in this highly characteristic location for an anterior temporal lobe perivascular space.

70.2 Correct: D. Adjacent to a branch of the middle cerebral artery.

A very helpful imaging characteristic for this entity is the proximity to a branch of the middle cerebral artery and associated focal cortical thinning or absence at the site of contact.

Other choices and discussion
A. In contrast to enlarged perivascular spaces in other locations, perilesional T2/FLAIR signal hyperintensity is common (80%) and certainly does not exclude the diagnosis.
B. Stability of size over time is expected.
C, E. The anterior temporal lobe perivascular space follows CSF intensity on the various MR sequences and accordingly does not enhance or restrict diffusion.

70.3 Correct: E. Inferior third of the basal ganglia.

The inferior third of the basal ganglia is the most common location in which enlarged perivascular spaces are encountered overall.

Other choices and discussion
D. The most common location for giant perivascular spaces (greater than 1.5 cm) in particular is the midbrain.
A–C. Enlarged perivascular spaces are less commonly seen in the subcortical white matter, dentate nucleus, and anterior temporal lobe.

References

Lim AT, Chandra RV, Trost NM, et al. Large anterior temporal Virchow-Robin spaces: unique MR imaging features. *Neuroradiology.* 2015;57(5):491–499.

Rawal S, Croul SE, Willinsky RA, et al. Subcortical cystic lesions within the anterior superior temporal gyrus: a newly recognized characteristic location for dilated perivascular spaces. *AJNR Am J Neuroradiol.* 2014;35(2):317-322.

Spine

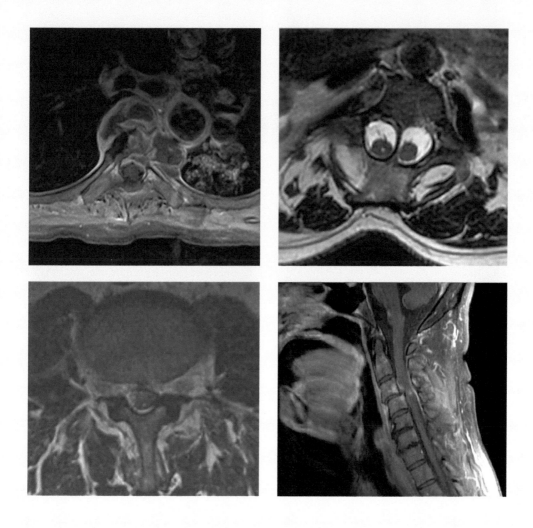

Case 71

Please refer to the following images to answer the next three questions:

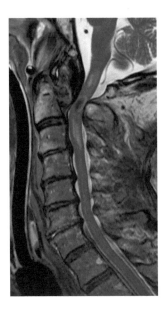 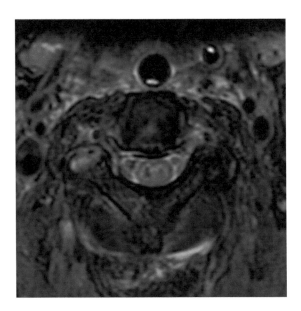

A 70 year-old-male who was found down and noted to have facial trauma presents for evaluation.

71.1 Which of the following statements regarding the fracture depicted in the above case is **TRUE**?

A. It has the highest rate of nonunion among fractures of its type.

B. It is caused by axial loading.

C. It is considered a stable fracture.

D. It constitutes greater than half of all C2 fractures.

E. It is referred to as a "Hangman's fracture."

71.2 What acute spinal cord injury is depicted in this case?

A. Contusion.

B. Hemorrhagic cord contusion.

C. Infarction.

D. Syrinx.

E. Transection.

71.3 Which of the following statements regarding cervical spine trauma is **TRUE**?

A. Adults are more likely than children to sustain traumatic spinal cord injury without radiographic abnormality (SCIWORA).

B. Improved neurologic outcomes are associated with surgical decompression greater than 24 hours following traumatic spinal cord injury.

C. Central cord syndrome most often occurs with hyperflexion injuries of the cervical spine.

D. The presence of cord hemorrhage in the setting of acute traumatic spinal cord injury is predictive of poor neurologic recovery.

E. Greater than half of all traumatic spinal cord injuries occur in the thoracic spine.

Answers and Explanations

71.1 Correct: A. It has the highest rate of nonunion among fractures of its type.

The fracture depicted in the above case is a type II dens (odontoid process) fracture. A type II dens fracture occurs at the base of the dens, separating it from the body of C2. This fracture is more difficult to treat and is more likely to result in nonunion than type I dens fractures (involving only the superior portion of the dens) and type III dens fractures (involving the body of C2 inferior to the base of the dens).

Other choices and discussion

B. A variety of mechanisms are responsible for this injury, including anterior-posterior and posterior-anterior translation and hyperflexion, but axial loading, which may produce burst fractures of the spinal column, is not one of the recognized mechanisms.
C. Type II dens fractures are considered to be unstable fractures.
D. Type II dens fractures constitute approximately one-third, and not one-half, of all C2 fractures.
E. A Hangman's fracture refers to traumatic spondylolisthesis of C2, not a type II dens fracture.

71.2 Correct: B. Hemorrhagic cord contusion.

There is focal T2 hypointense signal within the cord at the C2 level, representing intramedullary hemorrhage, surrounded by high-T2 signal, representing edema; these findings are compatible with hemorrhagic cord contusion.

Other choices and discussion

A. Simple contusion is not the best answer because hemorrhage is also present in the cord.
C. Infarction is incorrect as the injury in the question stem is mechanical in nature.
D. Syrinx can develop as a late complication of traumatic spinal cord injury and is not depicted in the above MR images.

E. While the cord has sustained trauma, no discontinuity in the cord is shown to suggest transection.

71.3 Correct: D. The presence of cord hemorrhage in the setting of acute traumatic spinal cord injury is predictive of poor neurologic recovery.

Several studies have shown that cord hemorrhage is associated with poor neurologic status on presentation, with patients more likely to have a complete spinal cord injury, and is also an independent poor prognostic indicator for neurologic recovery.

Other choices and discussion
The other choices are false.
A. Children, not adults, are more likely to sustain SCIWORA due to relatively greater ligamentous laxity.
B. Early (<24 hours) surgical decompression following traumatic spinal cord injury is associated with improved neurologic outcomes when compared to delayed surgical decompression.
C. Central cord syndrome most often occurs with hyperextension (not hyperflexion) injuries of the cervical spine.
E. Greater than half of all traumatic spinal cord injuries occur in the cervical spine.

References

Fehlings MG, Vaccaro A, Wilson JR, et al. Early versus delayed decompression for traumatic cervical spinal cord injury: results of the Surgical Timing in Acute Spinal Cord Injury Study (STASCIS). *PLoS One*. 2012;7(2):e32037.

Greene KA, Dickman CA, Marciano FF, et al. Acute axis fractures. Analysis of management and outcome in 340 consecutive cases. *Spine (Phila Pa 1976)*. 1997;22(16):1843–1852.

Miyanji F, Furlan JC, Aarabi B, et al. Acute Cervical Traumatic Spinal Cord Injury: MR Imaging Findings Correlated with Neurologic Outcome—Prospective Study with 100 *Consecutive Patients. Radiology*. 2007;243:820–827.

Case 72

Please refer to the following images to answer the next three questions:

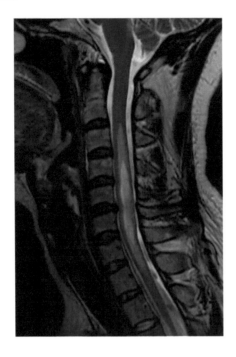 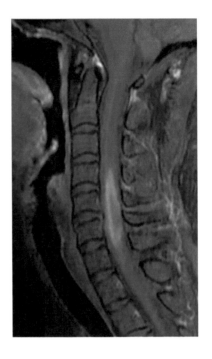

A 44-year-old female with a history of bilateral optic neuritis three months ago reports to the ER with new myelopathy progressing over the course of 3 days.

72.1 What is the **MOST** likely diagnosis based on the history and imaging findings?

A. Acute disseminated encephalomyelitis (ADEM).

B. Spinal cord ependymoma.

C. Spinal cord infarction.

D. Neuromyelitis optica spectrum disorder (NMOSD).

E. Multiple sclerosis (MS).

72.2 Which autoantibody is associated with NMOSD?

A. Anti-HU.

B. Anti-VGKC.

C. MOG-IgG.

D. Anti-GFAP.

E. AQP4-IgG.

72.3 Which of the following statements regarding neuromyelitis optica spectrum disorder (NMOSD) is **TRUE**?

A. Periependymal brain lesions are typical of NMOSD.

B. The detection of serum autoantibodies to aquaporin-4 (AQP4-IgG) is necessary for the diagnosis of NMOSD.

C. NMOSD occurs more frequently in men than in women.

D. Brain lesions oriented perpendicularly to the ventricles are typical for NMOSD.

E. Both optic neuritis and transverse myelitis are necessary for the diagnosis of NMOSD.

Answers and Explanations

72.1 Correct: D. Neuromyelitis optica spectrum disorder (NMOSD).

The MRI shows a longitudinally extensive (greater or equal to three vertebral segments) intramedullary lesion with ill-defined enhancement. Given the history of prior optic neuritis and new imaging findings compatible with acute myelitis, the most likely diagnosis is NMOSD. NMOSD is an autoimmune demyelinating disorder, targeting primarily the optic nerves and spinal cord.

Other choices and discussion

A. Acute disseminated encephalomyelitis is a postinfectious autoimmune disorder of the central nervous system (CNS) which can present with acute transverse myelitis, but is typically a monophasic illness, unlike the case presented here.

B. An intramedullary spinal cord ependymoma would not typically present subacutely, and the enhancement pattern should be more mass-like on imaging.

C. Spinal cord infarction presents acutely over the course of minutes to sometimes hours. Typical imaging findings include cord signal abnormality that preferentially involves the gray matter in the anterior cord ("owl's eyes" appearance). Enhancement can be seen in spinal cord infarct but occurs in the subacute (not acute) phase.

E. Typical cord lesions in multiple sclerosis are short segment (less than or equal to 1 vertebral segment).

72.2 Correct: E. AQP4-IgG.

Detectable serum antibodies to the water channel aquaporin-4 (AQP4-IgG) are highly specific for clinically diagnosed NMOSD.

Other choices and discussion

A, B. Anti-HU and Anti-VGKC are antibodies implicated in autoimmune encephalitis.

C. MOG-IgG is implicated in antimyelin oligodendrocyte glycoprotein (anti-MOG) syndromes, which have overlapping clinical and imaging features with, but are distinct from NMOSD.

D. Anti-GFAP mediates autoimmune glial fibrillary acidic protein (GFAP) astrocytopathy.

72.3 Correct: A. Periependymal brain lesions are typical of NMOSD.

Typical lesions of NMOSD reflect the distribution of AQP4 expression in the CNS. There is periependymal involvement of the hypothalamus, thalamus, corpus callosum, and brainstem periaqueductal region including the area postrema in the dorsal medulla (an area in the brainstem that plays a role in the control of autonomic functions including vomiting). Optic nerve and spinal cord involvement is also typical.

Other choices and discussion

B. The diagnosis of NMOSD can be made if testing for AQP4-IgG is negative or unavailable and if at least two core clinical characteristics of NMOSD are met. One of the core clinical features must be optic neuritis, acute myelopathy due to longitudinally extensive transverse myelitis, or area postrema syndrome (intractable hiccups, nausea, and vomiting) with corresponding MR findings.

C. NMOSD occurs more frequently in women.

D. Brain lesions oriented perpendicularly to the ventricles are seen in MS and are not usually seen in NMOSD.

E. If AQP4-IgG is detected, one core clinical characteristic (e.g., either optic neuritis or transverse myelitis) is sufficient for diagnosis.

References

Dutra BG, da Rocha AJ, Nunes RH, et al. Neuromyelitis optica spectrum disorders: spectrum of MR imaging findings and their differential diagnosis. *Radiographics*. 2018;38:169–193.

Wingerchuk DM, Banwell B, Bennett JL, et al. International consensus diagnostic criteria for neuromyelitis optic spectrum disorders. *Neurology*. 2015;85:177–189.

Case 73

Please refer to the following images to answer the next three questions:

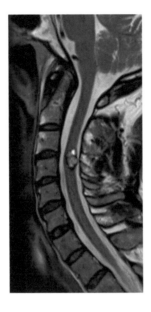 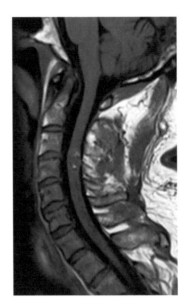

A 52-year-old male presents with slowly progressive arm and leg weakness.

73.1 What is the **MOST** likely diagnosis?

A. Spinal cord intramedullary metastasis.

B. Spinal dural arteriovenous fistula.

C. Spinal cord hemangioblastoma.

D. Spinal cord type II arteriovenous malformation (AVM).

E. Spinal cord cavernous malformation.

73.2 What type of lesion is depicted above, according to the Zabramski MRI classification system for cavernous malformations (CMs)?

A. Type I.

B. Type II.

C. Type III.

D. Type IV.

E. Type V.

73.3 Which of the following statements is **TRUE** regarding cavernous malformations (CMs)?

A. CMs are more frequently found in men than in women.

B. Arteriovenous shunting is a feature of CMs.

C. CMs do not enhance following contrast administration.

D. CMs can arise de novo.

E. Familial cavernous malformations are associated with developmental venous anomalies.

Answers and Explanations

73.1 Correct: E. Spinal cord cavernous malformation.

The MR images show an intramedullary lesion with a T2 hyperintense core and complete T2 hypointense rim consistent with a cavernous malformation; this appearance has been likened to a mulberry or popcorn. There is no surrounding edema.

Other choices and discussion

A. A spinal cord intramedullary metastasis would be expected to enhance and have perilesional edema.

B. A spinal dural arteriovenous fistula (type I spinal AVM) would exhibit prominent perimedullary flow voids and long-segment T2 signal abnormality with or without cord enhancement, reflecting arterialization of the perimedullary veins and resultant venous congestion and ischemia of the cord, respectively.

C. A discrete enhancing intramedullary nodule or mass in contact with the dorsal pial surface of the spinal cord with disproportionate cord edema or syrinx and perimedullary flow voids (in larger lesions) would be characteristic of spinal cord hemangioblastoma.

D. A type II spinal AVM or glomus-type AVM is composed of a discrete intramedullary nidus of tortuous, dilated vascular structures.

73.2 Correct: B. Type II.

Type II CMs are characterized by a reticulated mixed signal intensity core on both T1WI and T2WI, surrounded by a hypointense rim on T2WI and corresponding to areas of thrombosis and hemorrhage of varying ages surrounded by hemosiderin-stained neuronal tissue.

Other choices and discussion

C. Type III CMs are similar to Type 2 CMs but lack T1 hyperintensity within the core and reflect chronic resolved hemorrhage.

A. Type I CMs are characterized by a hyperintense core on T1WI and correspond to subacute hemorrhage.

D. Type IV CMs are seen as punctate lesions on gradient echo images.

E. Type V CMs are not part of the original Zabramski classification. The annual hemorrhage rate is significantly greater for type I and type II CMs than it is for type III and type IV CMs. CMs that have recently bled exhibit central T1 hyperintensity and perilesional edema. Following hemorrhage, a CM will evolve from type 1 to a type 2 or 3 appearance over the course of a year as long as there is no repeated hemorrhage.

73.3 Correct: D. CMs can arise de novo.

While most CMs are thought to be congenital, there is a relationship between central nervous system (CNS) irradiation and the development of CMs, particularly if the treatment was administered at a young age. Radiation-induced CMs present within the radiation port years to decades following treatment, where they are more likely to be multiple, and are more likely to hemorrhage compared to their sporadic counterparts. CMs have also been reported to arise in association with preexisting developmental venous anomalies.

Other choices and discussion

A. CMs are found more frequently in women than in men.

B. They are composed of endothelial-lined caverns and do not result in arteriovenous shunting.

C. Contrast enhancement is occasionally observed in cavernous CMs.

E. In contrast to sporadic CMs, familial CMs are unlikely to be associated with developmental venous anomalies.

References

Flemming KD, Kumar S, Lanzino G, et al. Baseline and Evolutionary Radiologic Features in Sporadic, Hemorrhagic Brain Cavernous Malformations. *AJNR Am J Neuroradiol.* 2019;40(6):967–972.

Jain R, Robertson PL, Gandhi D, et al. Radiation-induced cavernomas of the brain. *AJNR Am J Neuroradiol.* 2005;26(5):1158–1162.

Petersen TA, Morrison LA, Schrader RM, et al. Familial versus Sporadic Cavernous Malformations: Differences in Developmental Venous Anomaly Association and Lesion Phenotype. *AJNR Am J Neuroradiol.* 2010;31:377–382.

Case 74

Please refer to the following images to answer the next three questions:

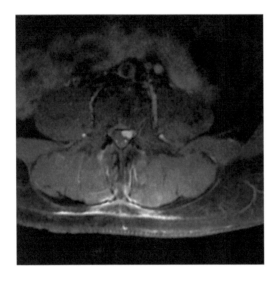
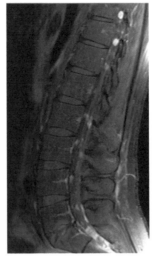
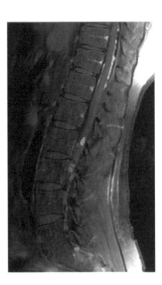

A 58-year-old female with history of breast cancer presents with progressive lower extremity weakness.

74.1 What is the **MOST** likely diagnosis?

A. Guillain-Barre syndrome.

B. Arachnoiditis ossificans.

C. Neurofibromatosis type II.

D. Leptomeningeal carcinomatosis.

E. Charcot-Marie-Tooth disease.

74.2 Which test or finding would confirm the diagnosis?

A. CSF cytology.

B. Albunimocytologic dissociation.

C. Genetic testing for Merlin mutation.

D. CSF xanthochromia.

E. CT of the lumbar spine.

74.3 Which imaging test is **MOST** sensitive for detection of leptomeningeal carcinomatosis?

A. Contrast-enhanced MRI.

B. CT myelography.

C. Fluorodeoxyglucose positron emission tomography (FDG PET).

D. In-111 cisternography.

E. Digital subtraction angiography (DSA).

Answers and Explanations

74.1   Correct: D. Leptomeningeal carcinomatosis.

Leptomeningeal carcinomatosis occurs as a result of cerebrospinal fluid (CSF) dissemination of a malignancy, either primary central nervous system (CNS) malignancy or extra-CNS cancer. The most common site is the lumbar spine. It may manifest as diffuse enhancement, coating the nerve roots and surface of the cord, multiple discrete enhancing nodules in the subarachnoid space, or a solitary enhancing mass.

Other choices and discussion

A. Guillain-Barre syndrome is a monophasic postinfectious autoimmune disorder involving the peripheral nervous system, presenting with ascending weakness. Smooth enhancement of the nerve roots, with predilection for the ventral nerve roots, is seen in GuillainBarré; nodular enhancement is not present.

B. Arachnoiditis ossificans is a rare complication of arachnoiditis with bone formation, which is better assessed on CT but enhancing nodules are not present.

C. Patients with neurofibromatosis type II may have multiple enhancing nodules in the cauda equina, either from multiple schwannomas and/or drop metastases from ependymoma. In this older patient with a breast cancer history, leptomeningeal spread of her known malignancy is more likely than a new diagnosis of NF-II, but neurofibromatosis can have a similar imaging appearance.

E. Charcot-Marie-Tooth, or hereditary motor and sensory neuropathy, is a group of genetic disorders which result in diffuse peripheral nerve enlargement and may involve the intraspinal nerve roots. Enhancement may be present but is usually not a prominent feature.

74.2   Correct: A. CSF cytology.

CSF analysis with cytology is highly specific for leptomeningeal carcinomatosis.

Other choices and discussion

B. Albunimocytologic dissociation, or elevation of CSF protein with increase in white blood cells, is characteristic of GuillainBarré syndrome.

C. Genetic testing for Merlin mutation is diagnostic of neurofibromatosis type II.

D. CSF xanthochromia is seen in subarachnoid hemorrhage.

E. CT of the lumbar spine may have a complimentary role in metastatic disease to assess the bones, but is not sensitive or specific for leptomeningeal disease.

74.3   Correct: A. Contrast-enhanced MRI.

Contrast-enhanced MRI is highly sensitive for the three patterns of leptomeningeal carcinomatosis: (1) "sugar coating" with diffuse enhancement along nerve roots and the surface of the cord, (2) multiple discrete enhancing nodules, and (3) solitary enhancing nodule.

Other choices and discussion

B. CT myelography may be helpful in patients who cannot undergo MRI to look for intrathecal filling defects, but is less sensitive and specific compared with MRI.

C. FDG PET may be positive with a large enough lesion burden, but small lesions (<1 cm) may be below the sensitivity of PET.

D, E. There is no role for In-111 cisternography and DSA for detection of leptomeningeal carcinomatosis.

References

Chapter 52 Leptomeningeal Carcinomatosis. In: Runge V, Morelli J, ed. Essentials of Clinical MR. 1st Edition. Thieme; 2010.

Chapter 15 Spinal Tumors. In: Naidich TP, Castillo M, Cha S, Smirniotopoulos, eds. Imaging of the Brain. Expert Radiology Series. Elsevier Saunders; 2013.

Case 75

Please refer to the following images to answer the next three questions:

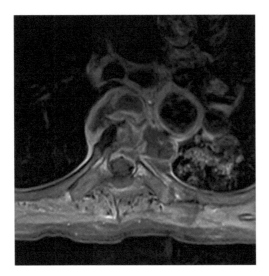

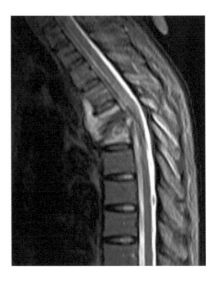

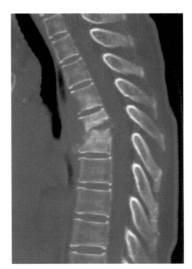

A 65-year-old female presents with two weeks of progressive back pain.

75.1 What is the **MOST** likely diagnosis?

A. Infectious spondylitis.

B. Osseous metastatic disease.

C. Neuropathic spinal arthropathy.

D. Aggressive hemangioma.

E. Aneurysmal bone cyst.

75.2 What imaging feature is **MOST** helpful to distinguish pyogenic spondylitis from tuberculous spondylitis?

A. Endplate irregularity.

B. Vertebral body enhancement.

C. Gas in the disc space.

D. Fluid collection in the paravertebral soft tissues.

E. Disc height loss.

75.3 What imaging feature is **MOST** helpful to distinguish infectiousspondylitis from an aggressive inflammatory or degenerative spondyloarthopathy?

A. Endplate irregularity.

B. Vertebral body enhancement.

C. Gas in the disc space.

D. Fluid collection in the paravertebral soft tissues.

E. Disc height loss.

Answers and Explanations

75.1 Correct: A. Infectious spondylitis.

The MRI and CT images show findings of infectious spondylitis, with destructive changes of the opposing endplates of T4-T5, vertebral body height loss, bone marrow edema, and focal kyphosis. In addition, there are multiple peripherally enhancing fluid collections in the surrounding paravertebral and epidural spaces consistent with abscesses.

Other choices and discussion

C. Given that the process is centered on the disc space, the primary differential consideration would be an aggressive destructive/degenerative process such as a neuropathic or Charcot joint; however, the presence of paravertebral abscesses strongly favors infection.

B, D, E. Processes that are centered in the bone rather than the disc space such as osseous metastatic disease, aggressive hemangiomas, and aneurysmal bone cysts may also have extraosseous extension. However, the paraspinal and epidural extension will not be as irregular and multiloculated in appearance as abscesses.

75.2 Correct: E. Disc height loss.

The above case is due to tuberculous spondylitis. Destruction of the vertebral body resulting in more than 50% height loss is more frequent (and severe) in tuberculous spondylitis than in pyogenic spondylitis.

Other choices and discussion

A, B, D. Tuberculous spondylitis shares many features with pyogenic spondylitis, including endplate irregularity, vertebral body enhancement, and fluid collections in the paravertebral soft tissues. Relative sparing of the disc space is more common with TB than with typical pyogenic organisms, and while this difference is suggestive, it is not entirely specific.

C. Gas in the disc space, or vacuum phenomenon is a feature of discogenic degenerative disease, not infection.

75.3 Correct: D. Fluid collection in the paravertebral soft tissues.

Degenerative disc disease, inflammatory arthropathy, and neuropathic spinal arthropathy share overlapping image features with infectious spondylitis, which can make accurate diagnosis difficult. The presence of significant paravertebral inflammatory changes or frank abscesses is rare in the absence of infection and is, therefore, helpful in making a more specific diagnosis.

Other choices and discussion

A, B, E. Endplate irregularity, vertebral body enhancement, and disc height loss are overlapping features that can be seen with degenerative disc disease, inflammatory arthropathy, and neuropathic spinal arthropathy.

C. While infection with gas-forming organisms may show gas within paravertebral abscesses, gas in the disc space itself almost always relates to vacuum disc phenomenon, a finding that is more specific for degenerative disc disease than for infection.

References

De Vuyst D, Vanhoenacker F, Gielen J, et al. Imaging features of musculoskeletal tuberculosis *Eur Radiol.* 2003;13:1809–1819.

Chang MC, Wu HTH, Lee CH, et al. Tuberculous spondylitis and pyogenic spondylitis: comparative magnetic resonance imaging features. *Spine.* 2006;31:782–788.

Case 76

Please refer to the following images to answer the next three questions:

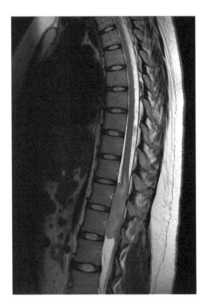 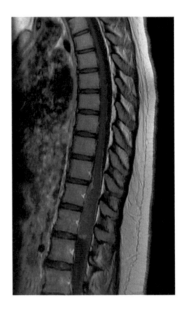

A 14-year-old female presents with progressive lower extremity weakness.

76.1 Where is the abnormality located?

A. Intradural intramedullary.

B. Intradural extramedullary.

C. Extradural extramedullary.

D. Osseous with extraosseous extension.

E. Paraspinal soft tissues

76.2 What is the **MOST** likely diagnosis?

A. Cord infarct.

B. Transverse myelitis.

C. Astrocytoma.

D. Ependymoma.

E. Dural arteriovenous fistula.

76.3 Which spinal cord tumor is **MOST** commonly associated with hemorrhage?

A. Astrocytoma.

B. Ependymoma.

C. Hemangioblastoma.

D. Lymphoma.

E. Metastasis.

Answers and Explanations

76.1 Correct: A. Intradural intramedullary.

The lesion is intradural and intramedullary, as it results in expansion and infiltration of the cord.

Other choices and discussion

B. Intradural extramedullary lesions maintain the normal dural margins, compress and displace the cord, and may result in cord edema but direct infiltration is uncommon.
C. Extradural extramedullary lesions compress the dura as well as the cord.
D. Osseous lesions with extraosseous extension may extend into the epidural space (which is extraduralextramedullary); no osseous abnormality is seen in this case.
E. This lesion arises from the spinal cord located within the spinal canal. There is no paraspinal soft tissue involvement on the provided images.

76.2 Correct: C. Astrocytoma.

The mass-like appearance of the lesion with associated cord expansion is helpful in determining this lesion to be neoplastic, as nonneoplastic etiologies are rarely so mass-like and expansile. The infiltrative T2 signal and mild enhancement without hemorrhage, peritumoral cysts, or syrinx formation best describes an astrocytoma.

Other choices and discussion

D. Ependymomas are more likely to have hemorrhage, peritumoral cysts, or an associated syrinx; however, there is an overlap in imaging features of astrocytoma and ependymoma, and tissue sampling is generally necessary for a definitive diagnosis. In this case, the final pathology was WHO grade III anaplastic astrocytoma.
A. Cord infarct acutely demonstrates restricted diffusion in the central cord, with T2 hyperintensity, enhancement, and mild expansion in the subacute phase.

B. Transverse myelitis is an inflammatory condition that results in a longitudinally extensive T2 hyperintense lesion in the cord, which often enhances. Cord expansion in transverse myelitis is typically mild if present.
E. Dural arteriovenous fistulae result in progressive T2 signal abnormality in the cord, with mild expansion related to venous congestion. Large flow voids from dilated venous collaterals are the key to this diagnosis.

76.3 Correct: B. Ependymoma.

Ependymomas are the most common spinal cord tumor to demonstrate hemorrhage on imaging. They are typically associated with the "cap sign," a low-T2 intensity rim around the mass, which is related to prior hemorrhage and is present in 20 to 33% of cases.

Other choices and discussion

A, D. Astrocytoma and lymphoma rarely hemorrhage.
C. Hemangioblastomas are vascular tumors which also hemorrhage and demonstrate a cap sign, although less commonly than ependymomas.
E. The risk of hemorrhage of an intramedullary metastasis depends on the tumor type but is overall less common than ependymoma.

References

Koeller KK, Rosenblum RS, Morrison AL. Neoplasms of the spinal cord and filum terminale: radiologic-pathologic correlation. *Radiographics*. 2000;20(6):1721–1749.

Lowe GM. Magnetic resonance imaging of intramedullary spinal cord tumors. *J Neurooncol*. 2000;47(3):195–210.

Case 77

Please refer to the following images to answer the next three questions:

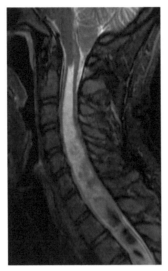

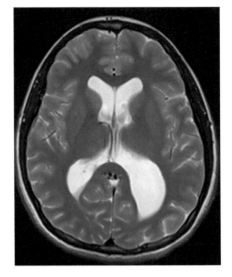

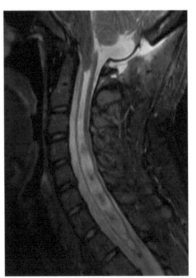

A 22-year-old female presents with headaches and extremity paresthesias.

77.1 Which of the following imaging findings **DO NOT** support the diagnosis of a Chiari I malformation?

A. Hydrocephalus.

B. Cerebellar tonsils lying 3 mm below foramen magnum.

C. Crowding at the craniocervical junction.

D. Cord syrinx.

E. Pointed morphology of the cerebellar tonsils.

77.2 What imaging technique can be obtained for pre-operative evaluation?

A. Phase contrast CSF flow study.

B. CT cervical spine.

C. Fast imaging employing steady-state acquisition (FIESTA) MRI sequence.

D. Myelogram.

E. CT head.

77.3 Which of the following developmental anomalies is **MOST** commonly associated with Chiari I?

A. Retroflexed odontoid process.

B. Klippel Feil syndrome.

C. Atlantooccipital assimilation.

D. Scoliosis.

E. Incomplete C1 ring ossification.

Answers and Explanations

77.1 Correct: B. Cerebellar tonsils lying 3 mm below foramen magnum.

The cutoff distance used to diagnose a Chiari I malformation is 5 mm for the cerebellar tonsils below the foramen magnum. Measurements should be made at midline on a sagittal.

Other choices and discussion

A, C–E. Measurements should ALWAYS be used in conjunction with the morphology of the tonsils (classically pointed or peg-shaped), and the presence of crowding and effacement of the cerebrospinal fluid (CSF) spaces at the craniocervical junction, and secondary signs of cord syrinx and hydrocephalus, in order to avoid overcalling this diagnosis.

77.2 Correct: A. Phase-contrast CSF flow study.

Phase-contrast CSF flow study is generally obtained in the preoperative setting for assessment of CSF flow dynamics at the craniocervical junction. Findings of disorganized and turbulent CSF flow with elevated peak systolic velocity and decreased flow through the foramen magnum may help in confirming the diagnosis of Chiari I, especially in unclear borderline cases.

Other choices and discussion

B–E. Since the anatomic obstruction is already evident on routine imaging, the remainder of the imaging techniques do not add any additional information and are incorrect.

77.3 Correct: D. Scoliosis.

Scoliosis can be seen in up to 50% of cases.

Other choices and discussion

A–C, E. The other developmental anomalies are also associated with Chiari I but are seen at a lesser frequency.

References

Lucchetta M, Cagnin A, Calderone M, et al. Syringomyelia associated with Chiari I malformation. *Neurol Sci.* 2009;30(6):525–526.

Novegno F, Caldarelli M, Massa A, et al. The natural history of the Chiari Type I anomaly. *J Neurosurg Pediatr.* 2008;2(3):179–187.

Case 78

Please refer to the following images to answer the next three questions:

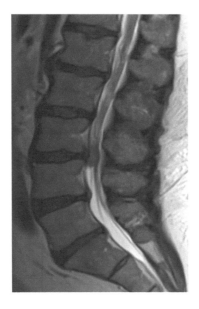 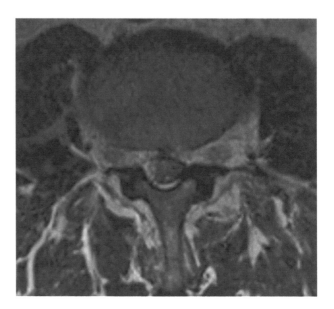

A 44-year-old male presents with back pain and radiculopathy.

78.1 What is the imaging finding?

A. Bone lesion.

B. Lesion within the spinal canal.

C. Acute fracture.

D. Discitis.

E. Hemorrhage.

78.2 Which of the following statements regarding disc herniations is **TRUE**?

A. Gas within the spinal canal related to disc vacuum phenomenon is a helpful clue in identifying intradural disc herniations.

B. 10% of disc extrusions are intradural.

C. MRI can always reliably distinguish intradural disc herniations from other lesions.

D. Disc protrusions are defined by craniocaudal migration.

E. Disc extrusions do not resolve spontaneously and require surgical intervention in the majority of cases.

78.3 Which of the following statements regarding discitisosteomyelitis is **TRUE**?

A. Noncontiguous level involvement is commonly seen in pyogenic osteomyelitis.

B. Intervertebral discs are typically spared in tuberculous osteomyelitis.

C. Type 2 Modic degenerative endplate changes can mimic discitis-osteomyelitis.

D. Soft-tissue calcifications are common in pyogenic infection.

E. Bone biopsy and blood cultures have similar diagnostic yield.

Answers and Explanations

78.1   Correct: B. Lesion within the spinal canal.

The images demonstrate a mildly T2 hyperintense lesion (relative to intervertebral disc signal) within the spinal canal. As the lesion insinuates between the cauda equina nerve roots, it appears ill-defined.

Other choices and discussion
A, C–E. No imaging findings are seen to suggest the other answer choices.

78.2   Correct: A. Gas within the spinal canal related to disc vacuum phenomenon is a helpful clue in identifying intradural disc herniations.

Intradiscal gas extending into the spinal canal can be a helpful clue in identifying intradural disc herniations when correlated with MRI.

Other choices and discussion
B–E. The other answer choices are incorrect. Intradural disc extrusions are very rare and are reportedly seen in only 0.3% of cases. Although MRI can be helpful, it may not always reliably distinguish focal extruded intradural disc fragments from other lesions, including disc herniations that have not traversed the posterior longitudinal ligament. Disc extrusions, not protrusions, are defined by prominent craniocaudal extension. The majority of disc extrusions resorb and resolve without surgical intervention; hence, they are medically managed.

78.3   Correct: B. Intervertebral discs are typically spared in tuberculous osteomyelitis.

Tuberculosis infects the vertebral bodies directly via hematogenous and lymphatic routes, typically spares the intervertebral discs, and spreads to contiguous and noncontiguous levels along the longitudinal ligaments.

Other choices and discussion
A. Noncontiguous, multilevel involvement is not commonly seen in pyogenic infection.
C. Type 1 (i.e., marrow edema), not type 2 (i.e., fatty marrow replacment), Modic degenerative endplate changes can mimic infection.
D. Soft-tissue calcifications associated with abscesses and phlegmon are associated with chronic granulomatous infections such as tuberculosis rather than pyogenic infection.
E. Although invasive, bone biopsies have a higher diagnostic yield compared to blood cultures.

Reference

Ross J, Moore K. Diagnostic imaging spine. Third edition. 2015.

Case 79

Please refer to the following images to answer the next three questions:

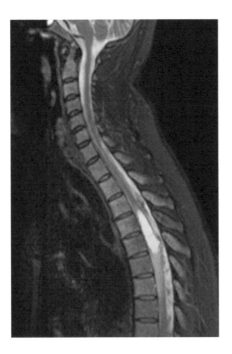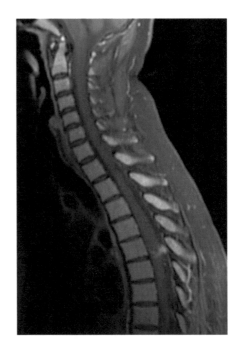

A 35-year-old male presents with left arm weakness and right leg paresthesia.

79.1   What is the **MOST** likely diagnosis?

A. Ependymoma.

B. Hemangioblastoma.

C. Metastasis.

D. Astrocytoma.

E. Cavernous malformation (CM).

79.2   What is the next **BEST** step in management?

A. Serial imaging.

B. Chemotherapy.

C. Immunotherapy.

D. Radiosurgery.

E. Angiogram.

79.3   Which of the following statements regarding hemangioblastomas is **TRUE**?

A. Most hemangioblastomas are completely intramedullary.

B. They can undergo malignant degeneration.

C. The majority of spinal hemangioblastomas occur sporadically.

D. They are WHO grade II tumors.

E. Cord edema does not improve after tumor resection.

Answers and Explanations

79.1 Correct: B. Hemangioblastoma.

The provided images show an avidly enhancing superficial mass along the dorsal aspect of the thoracic cord, with associated cyst/syrinx and regional prominent vascularity. Imaging findings are most consistent with a hemangioblastoma.

Other choices and discussion

C. Intramedullary metastatic disease is rare and unlikely in a young patient with no known history of malignancy.
E. Although similar imaging findings can be seen with an arteriovenous malformation, the above image features are not typical of a low-flow vascular lesion such as a CM, which usually does not enhance.
D. Astrocytomas are generally infiltrative lesions that demonstrate variable enhancement; the imaging findings in this case are not characteristic for this entity.
A. Spinal ependymomas are often well-circumscribed central cord lesions with peripheral hemosiderin staining.

79.2 Correct: E. Angiogram.

Given the hypervascular nature of the lesion and the presence of surrounding prominent vascular flow voids, digital subtraction angiography is the next best step for preoperative planning as well as potential arterial embolization.

Other choices and discussion

D. Radiosurgery can be considered in patients with small lesions or in the case of multiple lesions as seen in von Hippel-Lindau (VHL) syndrome.

A. Serial imaging is generally not appropriate when symptoms are present.
B, C. Chemotherapy (**B**) and immunotherapy (**C**) are not mainstay treatment options in hemangioblastoma, as surgical resection is typically curative.

79.3 Correct: C. The majority of spinal hemangioblastomas occur sporadically.

About 70% of hemangioblastomas occur sporadically and are solitary lesions; 30% of hemangioblastomas are associated with VHL syndrome and present as multiple cerebellar and cord lesions.

Other choices and discussion

B, D. Hemangioblastomas are slow-growing, benign WHO grade I tumors that do not undergo malignant degeneration.
A. Only 25% of hemangioblastomas are completely intramedullary, while the majority are surface lesions.
E. Cord edema tends to significantly improve after resection of the enhancing hypervascular tumor.

References

Deng X, Wang K, Wu L, et al. Intraspinal hemangioblastomas: analysis of 92 cases in a single institution: clinical article. *J Neurosurg Spine*. 2014;21(2):260–269.

Mechtler LL, Nandigam K. Spinal cord tumors: new views and future directions. *Neurol Clin*. 2013;31(1):241–268.

Case 80

Please refer to the following images to answer the next three questions:

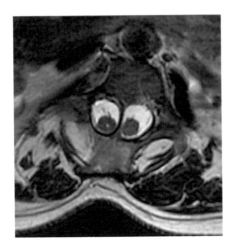 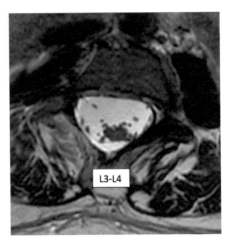

A 38-year-old female presents with leg pain and fasciculations.

80.1 What is the **MOST** likely diagnosis?

A. Diplomyelia.
B. Meningocele.
C. Dermal sinus tract.
D. Type I split cord malformation.
E. Type II split cord malformation.

80.2 What additional finding is present on these images?

A. Syrinx.
B. Dural ectasia.
C. Arachnoid web.
D. Bone lesion.
E. Arachnoiditis.

80.3 Split cord malformations are associated with which of the following?

A. Cephalocele.
B. Vertebral fusion anomaly.
C. Dermoid cyst.
D. A and B.
E. A, B, and C.

Answers and Explanations

80.1 Correct: D. Type I split cord malformation.

Split cord malformations are rare, accounting for 5% of all spinal dysraphisms. Type I split cord malformation, also known as diastematomyelia, is characterized by a duplicated cord and thecal sac, with the presence of a dividing short-segment fibroosseous spur, as seen in this case. There is fusion of the two hemicords, more caudally, as seen on the axial image.

Other choices and discussion
E. A type II malformation is characterized by a single dural sac containing both hemicords, with the lack of a fibroosseous spur. These malformations are associated with a low-lying tethered cord, which can lead to syrinx formation and hence be symptomatic. A tethered cord release procedure is the treatment of choice in these cases.
A. Diplomyelia is very rare and is seen in the presence of complete spinal canal duplication.
B, C. Meningocele or dermal sinus tract are not evident on these images.

80.2 Correct: B. Dural ectasia.

Prominent dural ectasia (patulous appearance of the spinal canal) is evident on the axial image.

Other choices and discussion
A. Although there is slight prominence of the central canal within one of the hemicords, it is felt to be within normal limits and does not represent a syrinx.
D. There is partial duplication of the spinous processes; however, no bone "lesion" is identified.
C, E. A fibroosseous spur related to the split cord malformation is present but no arachnoid web or imaging findings of arachnoiditis are seen.

80.3 Correct: E—A, B, and C.

Split cord malformations are associated with other spinal dysraphisms, vertebral fusion anomalies, scoliosis, meningoencephaloceles, dural ectasia, spinal lipoma, and dermoid cysts.

References

Alzhrani GA, Al-Jehani HM, Melancon D. Multi-level split cord malformation: do we need a new classification? *J Clin Imaging Sci.* 2014;24:4–32.

Ozturk E, Sonmez G, Mutlu H, et al. Split-cord malformation and accompanying anomalies. *J Neuroradiology.* 2008;35(3):150–156.

Case 81

Challenge

Please refer to the following images to answer the next three questions:

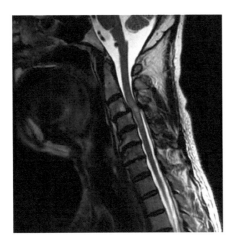 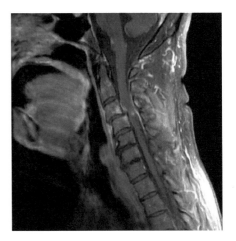

A 54-year-old male presents with progressive difficulty in walking and neck pain.

81.1 What is the **MOST** likely diagnosis based on the clinical history and imaging features?

A. Spinal dural arteriovenous fistula.

B. Neuromyelitis optica spectrum disorder.

C. Ependymoma.

D. Sarcoidosis.

E. Cervical spondylotic myelopathy.

81.2 The patient underwent surgical decompression for the presumed diagnosis of cervical spondylotic myelopathy and showed some clinical improvement. MRI performed 3 months following the surgery revealed adequate decompression but persistent cord enhancement. What is the next step in management?

A. Continued clinical follow-up.

B. Repeat MRI cervical spine with and without contrast in 6 months.

C. Brain MRI with and without contrast.

D. Lumbar puncture.

E. Spinal cord biopsy.

81.3 In what percentage of cases of cervical spondylotic myelopathy is contrast enhancement of the spinal cord seen?

A. Less than 15%.

B. 15 to 30%.

C. 30 to 50%.

D. 50 to 75%.

E. Greater than 75%.

Answers and Explanations

81.1 Correct: E. Cervical spondylotic myelopathy.

MRI shows severe spinal canal stenosis at the C3C4 level associated with cord compression, cord T2 signal abnormality, and short-segment contrast enhancement just below the level of maximal stenosis, typical of the enhancement seen in cervical spondylotic myelopathy (CSM). Contrast enhancement in CSM appears as a short-segment transverse or "pancake-like" band of enhancement just caudal to the level of maximal stenosis and within the region of T2 cord signal abnormality on sagittal images. On axial images, enhancement involves the white matter tracts along the periphery of the cord, with relative sparing of the central gray matter. Spinal cord enhancement in CSM occurs as a consequence of either increased vascular permeability from venous hypertension or formation of new vessels in response to injury. If moderate or severe spinal stenosis is absent or if there is deviation from the typical enhancement pattern of CSM, other differential diagnoses should be considered.

Other choices and discussion
A. A spinal dural arteriovenous fistula (SDAVF) is an abnormal connection between a spinal radiculomeningeal artery and a radicular vein, resulting in impaired venous drainage of the spinal cord, venous congestion, and subsequent myelopathy. The imaging triad of spinal cord edema, contrast enhancement, and dilated perimedullary vessels is suggestive of a SDAVF. The absence of perimedullary flow voids and the localized enhancement in the question stem argues against SDAVF. SDAVFs are also usually thoracolumbar in location.
B. Neuromyelitis optica spectrum disorder (NMOSD) is characterized by longitudinally extensive transverse myelitis, optic neuritis, and aquaporin-4 immunoglobulin G (AQP4 IgG) seropositivity, although not all features need to be present for diagnosis. Short-segment enhancement localized to the level of cervical spinal stenosis argues against this diagnosis.
C. Ependymoma is the most common primary tumor of the spinal cord in adults. It presents as a heterogeneous intramedullary mass and is frequently associated with tumoral cysts or syrinx and hemorrhage.

D. Sarcoidosis can present as an intramedullary lesion or as nodular leptomeningeal enhancement. When intramedullary in location, it can mimic longitudinally extensive transverse myelitis, which is seen in NMOSD, although the presence of central canal and dorsal subpial enhancement in sarcoidosis are potential discriminators.

81.2 Correct: A. Continued clinical follow-up.

Contrast enhancement in cervical spondylotic myelopathy persists for months to years following surgical decompression. In one study, enhancement was seen (but was often decreased) in 100% of cases between 3 and 12 months following decompression and in 75% of cases at 12 months following decompression.

Other choices and discussion
B. Unless there is clinical deterioration, repeat MRI of the cervical spine is not necessary.
C, D. Unless there is diagnostic uncertainty following surgical decompression and suspicion of a demyelinating or inflammatory cord lesion, further investigations with MRI of the brain with and without contrast or lumbar puncture are not indicated.
E. Spinal cord biopsy is not indicated here.

81.3 Correct: A. Less than 15%.

Gadolinium enhancement is seen in 7.3% of cases of cervical spondylotic myelopathy.

Other choices and discussion
B–E. The other responses state higher rates and are incorrect.

References

Flanagan EP, Krecke KN, Marsh RW, et al. Specific pattern of gadolinium enhancement in spondylotic myelopathy. *Ann Neurol.* 2014;76(1):54–65.

Wingerchuk DM, Banwell B, Bennett J, et al. International consensus diagnostic criteria for neuromyelitis optica spectrum disorders. *Neurology.* 2015;14;85(2):177–189.

Case 82

Challenge

Please refer to the following images to answer the next three questions:

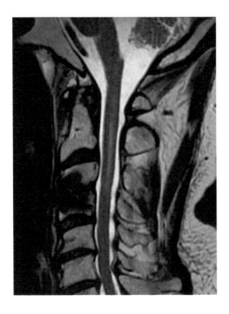
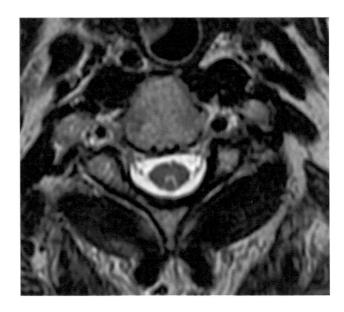

A 55-year-old male with history of cervical spinal stenosis at C3C4 initially presented with numbness and tingling in the hands. His symptoms improved following C3C4 anterior cervical discectomy and fusion. Postoperative imaging is shown above.

82.1 What is the **MOST** likely explanation for the imaging findings?

A. Spinal cord infarction.

B. Ependymoma.

C. Multiple sclerosis (MS).

D. Subacute combined degeneration.

E. Wallerian degeneration.

82.2 Which of the following is **NOT** in the differential diagnosis of signal abnormality involving the dorsal columns?

A. Vitamin B12 deficiency.

B. Nitrous oxide toxicity myelopathy.

C. Copper deficiency myelopathy.

D. Neurosyphilis.

E. Spinal dural arteriovenous fistula.

82.3 What signs and symptoms are expected with a lesion affecting the dorsal columns of the spinal cord?

A. Loss of pain and temperature sensation.

B. Loss of two-point discrimination, vibration, and proprioception.

C. Muscle atrophy and fasciculation.

D. Muscle weakness and increased tone.

E. Bowel and bladder dysfunction, and saddle anesthesia.

Answers and Explanations

82.1 Correct: E. Wallerian degeneration.

MRI shows T2 signal abnormality in the dorsal columns immediately superior to the C3C4 level, most likely due to chronic Wallerian degeneration because of prior cervical spondylotic myelopathy. Wallerian degeneration in the spinal cord is seen in the dorsal columns superior to and in the lateral columns inferior to the level of injury. This is manifested on MRI as hyperintense T2 signal in the affected tracts.

Other choices and discussion

A. Signal abnormality due to spinal cord infarction, in contrast, is situated in the gray matter centrally within the spinal cord, which is most susceptible to ischemia. Imaging findings of spinal cord infarction include hyperintense T2 signal, with restricted diffusion centrally within the spinal cord, which may have a "snake-eye" or "owl-eye" configuration on axial images. Sudden onset of symptoms would also support the diagnosis of spinal cord infarction.

B. An ependymoma is a space-occupying mass; the lesion in this case symmetrically involves the dorsal columns and does not exhibit mass effect.

C. Demyelinating plaques of MS in the spinal cord tend to be peripherally located (in the white matter) and tend to involve short segments of the cord, unlike the lesion in this case.

D. While subacute combined degeneration in the spinal cord secondary to vitamin B12 deficiency manifests on MRI as a hyperintense T2 signal in the dorsal columns and lateral columns, long-segment involvement of the cord is more typical. Also, this history of cervical myelopathy indicates that Wallerian degeneration is a better answer choice.

82.2 Correct: E. Spinal dural arteriovenous fistula.

Spinal dural arteriovenous fistulas can produce venous congestion in the spinal cord, which is manifested by swelling, T2 hyperintense signal, and enhancement. Engorged perimedullary veins can be seen on T2-weighted imaging as serpiginous signal voids in the subarachnoid space.

Other choices and discussion

A. MR images of subacute combined degeneration demonstrate T2 signal in the dorsal and lateral columns. Symmetric dorsal column involvement produces an "inverted V" appearance on axial images.

B. Nitrous oxide (NO) toxicity myelopathy can occur with prolonged use of NO in anesthesia or with NO abuse. The effect may be potentiated in patients with vitamin B12 deficiency. The MRI appearance can be indistinguishable from subacute combined degeneration.

C. Copper deficiency myelopathy can produce a clinical and radiographic syndrome indistinguishable from subacute combined degeneration.

D. Tabes dorsalis is a late manifestation of untreated neurosyphilis. MRI demonstrates T2 hyperintensity in the dorsal columns and cord atrophy.

82.3 Correct: B. Loss of two-point discrimination, vibration, and proprioception.

The dorsal column is part of an ascending pathway that is important for fine touch, conscious proprioception, and vibration.

Other choices and discussion

A. Loss of pain and temperature sensation would be seen in a lesion in the spinothalamic tract.

C. Choice muscle atrophy and fasciculation would be seen in a lesion involving the ventral (anterior) horn cells.

D. Muscle weakness and increased tone would be seen in a lesion involving the lateral corticospinal tract.

E. Bowel and bladder dysfunction, and saddle anesthesia, would be seen in cauda equina syndrome.

References

Becerra JL, Puckett WR, Hiester ED, et al. MR-pathologic comparisons of Wallerian degeneration in spinal cord injury. *AJNR Am J Neuroradiol.* 1995;16:125–133.

Valencia MP, Castillo M. MRI findings in post-traumatic spinal cord Wallerian degeneration. *Clin Imaging.* 2006;30:431–433.

Weidauer S, Nichtweiss M, Lanfermann H, et al. Spinal cord infarction: MR imaging and clinical features in 16 cases. *Neuroradiology.* 2002;44:851–857.

Case 83

Challenge

Please refer to the following images to answer the next three questions:

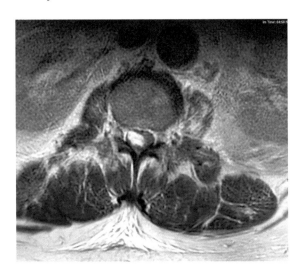 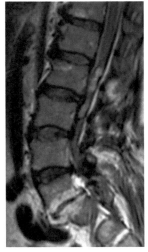 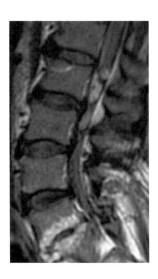

A 50-year-old male with history of recent endovascular repair of abdominal aortic aneurysm and lumbar drain placement presents with new lower extremity weakness. A recent prior MRI only showed L5S1 degenerative changes.

83.1 Where is the abnormality located?

A. Intradural intramedullary.

B. Intradural extramedullary.

C. Extradural extramedullary.

D. Osseous with extraosseous extension.

E. Paraspinal soft tissues.

83.2 What is the **MOST** likely diagnosis?

A. Intradural hematoma.

B. Epidural hematoma.

C. Subdural empyema.

D. Epidural abscess.

E. Myxopapillary ependymoma.

83.3 In what range does the conus medullaris normally terminate?

A. Mid T10–upper L1.

B. Mid T11–upper L2.

C. Mid T12–upper L3.

D. Mid L1–upper L4.

E. Mid L2–upper L5.

Answers and Explanations

83.1 Correct: B. Intradural extramedullary.

An irregular T2 hyperintense lesion with peripheral hypointense rim is present within the spinal canal from the L2L3 disc space to mid-L4 level. The axial image shows the lesion to be within the thecal sac rather than having mass effect on the dura (intradural). In addition, the lesion is outside of the spinal cord, as the conus terminates just above the lesion at the mid-L2 level (extramedullary). Therefore, the lesion is located within the intradural, extramedullary space.

Other choices and discussion

A, C. As stated above, the lesion is within the thecal sac (intradural) and outside of the cord (extramedullary), making choices (**A**) and (**C**) incorrect.

D. The lesion is not centered in the bone.

E. The lesion is not centered in the paraspinal soft tissues.

83.2 Correct: A. Intradural hematoma.

The intradural lesion is lobulated and T2 hyperintense, which suggests a fluid collection. The peripheral hypointensity is related to susceptibility from blood products and best fits the diagnosis of hematoma which was proven during surgery. The hematoma was likely a complication of lumbar drain placement, which was placed preoperatively to decrease cerebrospinal fluid (CSF) pressure during aortic aneurysm repair.

Other choices and discussion

C. Superinfection of this hematoma cannot be excluded based on imaging alone; however, a subdural empyema is typically more lobulated along the periphery of the spinal canal and would not be expected to have marked peripheral T2 hypointensity.

B, D. Epidural hematoma and epidural abscess are excluded based on the location of the lesion as discussed above.

E. A myxopapillary ependymoma could look similar on T2-weighted images as the tumor may hemorrhage; however, no abnormality was seen on a recent prior MRI, so a neoplasm would not be likely to arise in the short interval. In the absence of prior imaging, gadolinium-enhanced imaging may be helpful in distinguishing a myxopapillary ependymoma or other neoplasm from hematoma, as the former often shows areas of solid enhancement and the latter will either not enhance or show a thin peripheral rim of reactive enhancement.

83.3 Correct: C. Mid T12–upper L3.

The conus medullaris normally terminates near the lower L1 level and within the range of mid T12–upper L3. Knowing the normal location of the conus is important for determining if the cord is low-lying or tethered, and if the cord is abnormally high in the setting of caudal regression or for lumbar puncture planning. The other answers are incorrect.

Other choices and discussion

A, B, D, E: The other answers are incorrect because, as stated above, the conus typically terminates from T12 to L3.

References

Boukobza M, Haddar D, Boissonet M, et al. Spinal subdural haematoma: a study of three cases. *Clin Radiol.* 2001;56(6):475–480.

Kim JT, Bahk JH, Sung J. Influence of age and sex on the position of the conus medullaris and Tuffier's line in adults. *Anesthesiology.* 2003;99:1359–1363.

Pierce JL, Donahue JH, Nacey NC, et al. Spinal hematomas: what a radiologist needs to know. *Radiographics.* 2018;38(5):1516–1535.

Case 84

Challenge

Please refer to the following images to answer the next three questions:

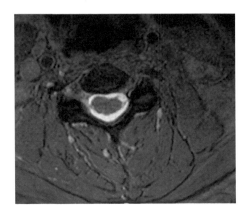 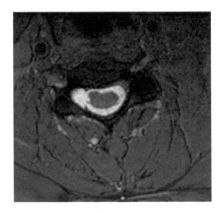

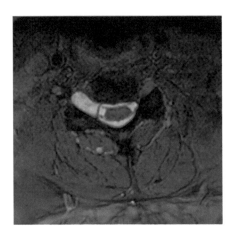

A 54-year-old male with remote history of motorcycle crash years presents with persistent right arm weakness.

84.1 What is the **MOST** likely diagnosis?

A. Meningeal diverticulum.

B. Schwannoma.

C. Neurofibroma.

D. Neuroma and pseudomeningocele.

E. Synovial cyst.

84.2 What level of the brachial plexus is affected in the provided images?

A. Roots.

B. Divisions.

C. Branches.

D. Trunks.

E. Cords.

84.3 What is the correct order of the brachial plexus?

A. Roots, divisions, branches, trunks, cords.

B. Roots, trunks, divisions, cords, branches.

C. Roots, cords, trunks, divisions, branches.

D. Roots, divisions, cords, trunks, branches.

E. Roots, branches, trunks, divisions, cords.

Answers and Explanations

84.1   Correct: D. Neuroma and pseudomeningocele.

Axial T2 images of the cervical spine show a fluid intensity lesion in the right C5C6 neural foramen. More subtly, there is a rounded "mass" along the right ventrolateral surface of the spinal cord, and the normal ventral nerve rootlets are not seen. These findings are a result of nerve root avulsion injury, with retraction of the avulsed nerve roots and the formation of a posttraumatic neuroma along the cord. Injury of the dura results in a pseudomeningocele containing cerebrospinal fluid (CSF) which is not contained by the meninges. This is an uncommon and severe formation of traumatic brachial plexus injury. Diagnosis of avulsion injury in the acute phase is essential to identify patients who may benefit from surgical intervention, with improvement in motor function.

Other choices and discussion

A. A meningeal diverticulum is a CSF-containing outpouching from the thecal sac which is lined by meninges. These are common incidental findings which typically occur at the cervicothoracic junction, but may also be seen in patients with spontaneous CSF leaks.

B, C. Benign peripheral nerve sheath tumors such as schwannomas and neurofibromas may be associated with the nerve roots in the neural foramen. Determining that the T2 hyperintensity in the neural foramen is a CSF collection and identifying the avulsed nerve roots are essential to distinguishing neuroma and pseudomeningocele from a nerve sheath tumor.

E. Synovial cysts are round cystic lesions that project from a joint space and are related to degenerative change of the spine.

84.2   Correct: A. Roots.

The nerve roots are the most proximal component of the peripheral nerve and directly exit the spinal cord. Ventral nerve roots contain motor fibers, and dorsal nerve roots, sensory fibers. Ventral nerve roots are avulsed in this case.

Other choices and discussion

B–E. The other answer choices are incorrect.

Since the lesion in this question is very proximal, answer choices **B** to **E** are incorrect. Divisions (**B**), branches (**C**), trunks (**D**), and cords (**E**) occur distal to the dorsal root ganglion.

84.3   Correct: B. Roots, trunks, divisions, cords, branches.

The mnemonic "Rad Techs Drink Cold Beer" may be helpful in remembering the components of the brachial plexus in order from proximal to distal: **R**oots, **T**runks, **D**ivisions, **C**ord, and **B**ranches. Each component can be visualized on MRI of the brachial plexus, and understanding the structure and function of the brachial plexus is essential for accurate interpretation.

Other choices and discussion

A, C–E. These answer choices do not correctly order the subdivisions of the brachial plexus: roots, trunks, divisions, cords, and branches.

References

Hayashi N, Yamamato S, Okubo T, et al. Avulsion injury of cervical nerve roots: enhanced intradural nerve roots at MR imaging. *Radiology*.1998;206(3):817–822.

Yoshikawa T, Hayashi N, Yamamoto S, et al. Brachial plexus injury: clinical manifestations, conventional imaging findings, and the latest imaging techniques. *Radiographics*. 2006;26(1 Suppl):S133–S143.

Case 85

Challenge

Please refer to the following images to answer the next three questions:

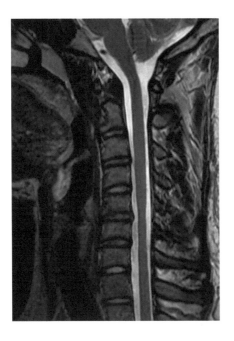 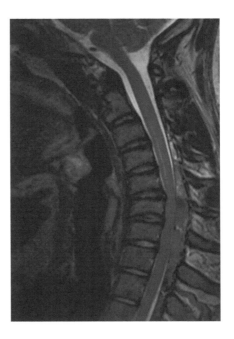

A 24-year-old female with progressive upper extremity symptoms.

85.1 What is the **MOST** likely diagnosis?

A. Giant cell tumor.

B. Schwannoma.

C. Epidural angiolipoma.

D. Hirayama disease.

E. Meningioma.

85.2 What is the **MOST** likely clinical presentation?

A. Hand muscular atrophy.

B. Upper and lower motor neuron symptoms.

C. Paresthesias.

D. Loss of sensation in a dermatomal pattern.

E. Ascending lower limb atrophy.

85.3 Which of the following statements regarding Hirayama disease is **TRUE**?

A. Also called adult-onset spinal muscular atrophy.

B. Characterized by progressive peripheral to central muscular atrophy.

C. Cord compression results from neck extension.

D. Findings stabilize after steady progression without clinical intervention.

E. Patients present with sensory symptoms.

Answers and Explanations

85.1 Correct: D. Hirayama disease.

The first image in neutral positioning demonstrates moderate cord atrophy, spanning the C5–7 levels. Upon flexion (second image), there is a large heterogenous dorsal epidural lesion compressing the C5–7 cord. This lesion demonstrated enhancement on postcontrast imaging (not included). Imaging findings are diagnostic of Hirayama disease. Although the etiology is controversial, the dominant opinion is that there is disproportionately decreased growth of the dura in relation to the vertebral column, causing a tight canal with flexion. Length of the cervical canal normally increases with flexion but in patients with Hirayama, the dural sac is unable to compensate, leading to engorgement of the epidural venous plexus and causing anterior shift and cord compression.

Other choices and discussion

A–C, E: While a dorsal epidural lesion is present on the flexion image, it is not present on the neutral image. Masses such giant cell tumor (**A**), schwannoma (**B**), angiolipoma (**C**), and meningioma (**D**) will not disappear with different positioning.

85.2 Correct: A. Hand muscular atrophy.

Repeated trauma from flexion eventually leads to necrosis of the C5–T1 anterior horn cells within the cord, which manifests as hand and forearm atrophy.

Other choices and discussion

B. Upper and lower motor neuron symptoms are present in patients with amyotropic lateral sclerosis.
E. Ascending lower limb atrophy is seen in Charcot–Marie–Tooth disease.

C, D. Patients with Hirayama do not classically present with sensory symptoms.

85.3 Correct: D. Findings stabilize after steady progression without clinical intervention.

Hirayama disease typically has an insidious onset and presents with upper extremity weakness and muscular atrophy in the C5–T1 distribution, involving the hands and forearms. Unilateral weakness and atrophy is more common than bilateral. Findings of Hirayama disease eventually stabilize after steady progression without clinical intervention.

Other choices and discussion

A. Hirayama disease is also called juvenile spinal muscular atrophy, since symptoms usually start in the teenage years.
B. Hirayma disease is not associated with truncal (central) or lower limb atrophy.
C. Cord compression results from repeated neck flexion, not extension.
E. Patients with Hirayama disease do not classically present with sensory symptoms.

References

Boruah DK, Prakash A, Gogoi BB, et al. The Importance of Flexion MRI in Hirayama Disease with Special Reference to Laminodural Space Measurements. *AJNR Am J Neuroradiol.* 2018;39(5):974–980.

Lehman VT, Luetmer PH, Sorenson EJ, et al. Cervical spine MR imaging findings of patients with Hirayama disease in North America: a multisite study. *AJNR Am J Neuroradiol.* 2013;34(2):451–6.

Head and Neck

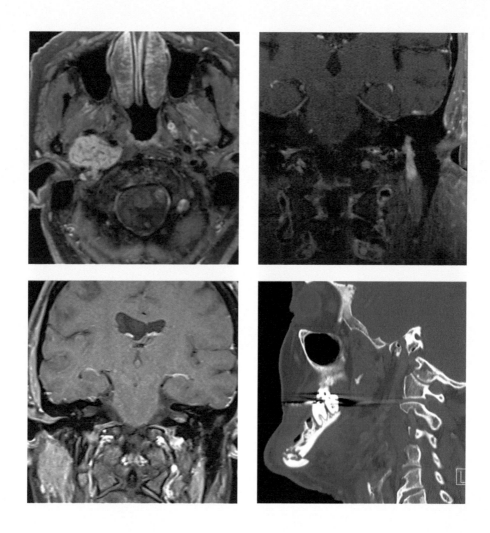

Case 86

Please refer to the following images to answer the next three questions:

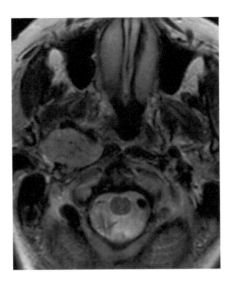
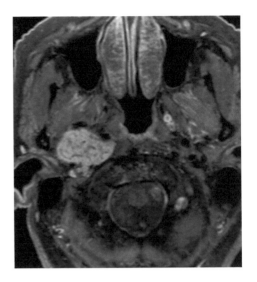

A 78-year-old female with hearing loss and rhythmic pulsing in the ear.

86.1 What is the **MOST** likely diagnosis for the above lesion arising from the jugular foramen?

A. Chondrosarcoma.

B. Schwannoma.

C. Paraganglioma.

D. Meningioma.

E. Metastasis.

86.2 Vascular supply of glomus jugulare is predominantly from the:

A. Superior thyroid artery.

B. Ascending pharyngeal artery.

C. Lingual artery.

D. Facial artery.

E. Maxillary artery.

86.3 Paragangliomas typically occur in association with all of the following syndromes **EXCEPT**:

A. Multiple endocrine neoplasia type 1 (MEN 1).

B. Multiple endocrine neoplasia type 2 (MEN 2).

C. Von Hippel-Lindau (VHL).

D. Neurofibromatosis type 1 (NF-1).

E. CarneyStratakis syndrome.

Answers and Explanations

86.1 Correct: C. Paraganglioma.

The above case shows a circumscribed hyperintense T2 mass with intrinsic flow voids, and marked enhancement in the right jugular foramen and carotid space. The hypervascular and "salt and pepper" appearance of this mass (the latter due to the presence of flow voids) emanating from the jugular foramen on MRI is most consistent with a paraganglioma (glomus jugulare), which is a benign but locally aggressive tumor arising from neural crest progenitor cells in and around the jugular foramen. In 4% of cases, these lesions can transform into malignant tumors with the potential for metastatic spread. They can be either sporadic or familial. On CT, paragangliomas present with permeative and lytic bony destruction of the margins of the jugular foramen, often with erosion of the jugular spine. They also tend to extend along pathways of least resistance, often superolaterally through the floor of the middle ear and into the hypotympanum and mastoid air cells.

Other choices and discussion

A. Chondrosarcomas are markedly T2 hyperintense masses without internal flow voids, which are present in the above lesion.
B. Jugular foramen schwannomas present with smooth remodeling and enlargement of the jugular foramen and are typically avascular or hypovascular relative to paragangliomas. Intrinsic flow voids are not usually present as in the above case.
D. Meningiomas frequently present with limited lytic or sclerotic changes of the bony margins of the jugular foramen and have characteristic dural "tails," a feature that is absent in the above case.
E. While a metastasis can also have destructive bony changes of the margins of the jugular foramen, the above homogeneously enhancing mass with intrinsic flow voids in a patient without a history of cancer is most consistent with a paraganglioma. Also, the clinical onset of symptoms is more rapid with metastasis than with paraganglioma, schwannoma, or meningioma.

86.2 Choice B. Ascending pharyngeal artery.

The main arterial supply for these vascular tumors is from the ascending pharyngeal artery, a branch of the external carotid artery. However, other branches of the external carotid artery, vertebral artery, and internal carotid artery may also contribute supply to these lesions. Digital subtraction angiography often shows a markedly hypervascular mass with enlarged feeding arteries, rapid and persistent tumor blush, and early draining veins.

Other choices and discussion

A. The superior thyroid artery is a branch of the external carotid artery that supplies the larynx and thyroid gland.

C. The lingual artery is a branch of the external carotid artery that supplies the oral floor and tongue.
D. The facial artery is a branch of the external carotid artery that supplies blood to structures of the face.
E. The maxillary artery is the larger of two terminal branches of the external carotid artery (the other being the superficial temporal artery) and supplies the deep structures of the face.

86.3 Correct: A. Multiple endocrine neoplasia type 1 (MEN1).

Parathyroid tumors, pancreatic islet cell tumors, and pituitary tumors are characteristic of MEN1. Other tumors associated with MEN1 include carcinoid tumors, lipomas, facial angiofibromas, adrenal cortical lesions, thyroid adenomas, pheochromocytomas, meningiomas, and leiomyomas. Paragangliomas do not typically occur in association with MEN1.

Other choices and discussion

B. MEN2 has three subtypes: MEN2A, MEN2B, and familial medullary thyroid cancer (FMTC). While MEN2A and MEN2B are associated with an increased risk of parathyroid hyperplasia and/or adenoma compared to FMTC, all three subtypes confer a risk of medullary thyroid cancer. Other lesions associated with MEN2 include pheochromocytomas, paragangliomas, and mucosal neuromas.
C. Lesions of VHL include central nervou system (CNS) hemangioblastomas, retinal hemangioblastomas, endolymphatic sac tumors, renal lesions such as renal cell carcionomas, cysts, and angiomyolipomas, pheochromocytomas, pancreatic lesions such as cysts and islet cell tumors, hepatic cysts, cystadenoma of the epididymis, and paragangliomas.
D. Tumor lesions of NF-1 include benign and malignant peripheral nerve sheath tumors, plexiform neurofibromas, optic nerve gliomas, pheochromocytomas, Wilms tumor, rhabdomyosarcoma, renal angiomyolipoma, carcinoid tumors, leiomyomas, and paragangliomas.
E. Lesions associated with CarneyStratakis syndrome, a syndrome with autosomal dominant inheritance, include paragangliomas and gastrointestinal stromal tumors.

References

Caldemeyer KS, Mathews VP, Azzarelli B, et al. The jugular foramen: a review of anatomy, masses, and imaging characteristics. *Radiographics*. 1997;17:1123–1139.

Fayad JN, Keles B, Brackmann DE. Jugular foramen tumors: clinical characteristics and treatment outcomes. *Otol Neurol*. 2010;31:299–305.

Lips C, Lentjes E, Hoppener J, et al. Familial paragangliomas. *Hered Cancer Clin Pract*. 2006;4:169–176.

Case 87

Please refer to the following images to answer the next three questions:

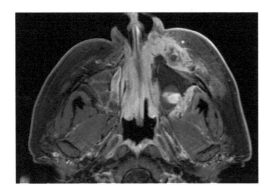
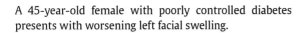
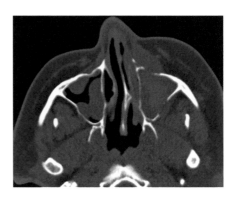

A 45-year-old female with poorly controlled diabetes presents with worsening left facial swelling.

87.1   What is the **MOST** likely diagnosis?

A. Squamous cell carcinoma.

B. Lymphoma.

B. Wegener's granulomatosis.

D. Allergic fungal sinusitis.

E. Acute invasive fungal sinusitis.

87.2   Which organism is responsible for most cases of acute invasive fungal sinus infections in immunocomprised patients with severe neutropenia?

A. Rhizopus.

B. Rhizomucor.

C. Absidia.

D. Mucor.

E. Aspergillus.

87.3   Which complication of acute invasive fungal sinusitis is the highest predictive indicator for mortality?

A. Cavernous sinus thrombosis.

B. Intracranial spread.

C. Internal carotid artery occlusion.

D. Mycotic aneurysm formation.

E. Cranial nerve involvement.

Answers and Explanations

87.1 Correct: E. Acute invasive fungal sinusitis.

In the above case, there is an ill-defined, irregular, and enhancing mass in the left maxillary sinus, most notably along the periphery, with involvement of the perimaxillary soft tissues including the retroantral fat (first image). As seen on CT, the mass destroys the anterior and posterolateral walls of the maxillary sinus (second image). Notably, the round enhancing structure in the maxillary sinus (first image) represents a concomitant polyp. Given the imaging findings of an aggressive and enhancing lesion with ill-defined margins in the paranasal sinuses and infiltration of the surrounding soft tissues in the setting of a diabetic patient, acute invasive fungal sinusitis is the most likely diagnosis. Acute invasive fungal sinusitis is a rapidly progressive infection, occurring primarily in patients with neutropenia, specifically those who are immuocompromised (e.g., individuals with leukemia, bone marrow transplant, AIDS, or on chronic immunosuppressive therapy) and those with poorly controlled diabetes. It is the most fatal form of fungal sinusitis with a mortality rate of 50 to 80%. Features of angioinvasion and hematogenous dissemination are commonly present. Endoscopic evaluation and tissue biopsy may be necessary to establish a definitive diagnosis.

Other choices and discussion

A. While the above findings of an ill-defined enhancing lesion with associated bony destruction can be seen with squamous cell carcinoma, a focal and irregular soft tissue mass can usually be identified. Also, the classic scenario for squamous cell carcinoma is a male patient older than 40 years old, who presents with symptoms of sinusitis refractory to medical therapy. In difficult cases, definitive diagnosis depends on tissue sampling.
B. As with squamous cell carcinoma, sinonasal lymphoma usually presents with a discrete soft tissue mass that diffusely and homogeneously enhances, although it can present as a diffusely infiltrating lesion along the walls of the paranasal sinuses. There is a greater predilection for involvement of the nasal cavity than the paranasal sinuses. In this case, the history of a diabetic patient with progressive symptoms should clue the reader into acute invasive fungal infection. In challenging cases, definitive diagnosis is based on tissue sampling.
C. Sinonasal Wegener's granulomatosis typically presents as nodular and destructive soft tissue masses centered in the nasal cavity, with associated chronic inflammatory changes, periantral soft tissue infiltration, and orbital extension. Nasal septal perforation is common. Imaging features often overlap with sinonasal lymphoma and

sarcoidosis. While this condition is generally indolent in contrast to acute invasive fungal sinusitis, it may transition to fulminating disease. Surgical confirmation may be needed for definitive diagnosis in specific cases.
D. Allergic fungal sinusitis does not typically present as a destructive mass. It is typically a disease of young atopic patients. Involvement of the nasal cavity as well as multiple and bilateral sinuses containing hyperattenuating material on CT is classic. Differential considerations for hyperdensity in the paranasal sinuses include inspissated secretions, fungal elements related to allergic fungal sinusitis or mycetoma, and blood.

87.2 Correct: E. Aspergillus.

Aspergillus species are responsible for up to 80% of acute invasive fungal sinus infections in immunocomprised patients with severe neutropenia, including those with hematologic malignancy or AIDS, and those undergoing bone marrow transplantation or receiving immunosuppressive therapy.

Other choices and discussion

A–D. Fungi of the Zygomycetes order including *Rhizopus*, *Rhizomucor*, *Absidia*, and *Mucor* are responsible for up to 80% of infections in patients with poorly controlled diabetes, particularly those with diabetic ketoacidosis.

87.3 Correct: B. Intracranial spread.

Intracranial involvement such as leptomeningeal enhancement predicts higher morbidity and mortality, with death occurring in greater than 70% of patients.

Other choices and discussion

A, C–E. While the other answer choices are complications of acute invasive fungal sinusitis, they are not the highest predictive indicator for mortality.

References

Aribandi M, McCoy VA, Bazan C 3rd. Imaging features of invasive and noninvasive fungal sinusitis: a review. *Radiographics*. 2007;27:1283–1296.

Groppo ER, El-Sayed IH, Aiken AH, et al. Computed tomography and magnetic resonance imaging characteristics of acute invasive fungal sinusitis. *Arch Otolaryngol Head Neck Surg*. 2011;137:1005–1010.

Middlebrooks EH, Frost CJ, De Jesus RO, et al. Acute invasive fungal rhinosinusitis: a comprehensive update of CT findings and design of an effective diagnostic imaging model. *AJNR Am J Neuroradiol*. 2015;36:1529–1535.

Case 88

Please refer to the following images to answer the next three questions:

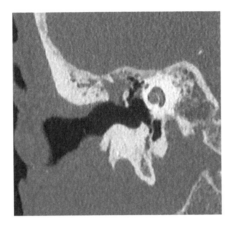

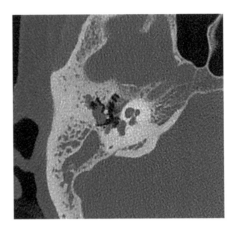

History withheld.

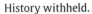

88.1 What is the **MOST** likely diagnosis?

A. Glomus tympanicum paraganglioma.

B. Pars flaccida cholesteatoma.

C. Chronic otitis media.

D. Cholesterol granuloma.

E. Congenital cholesteatoma.

88.2 Which MRI sequence is **MOST** useful in making a specific diagnosis of cholesteatoma?

A. Postcontrast fat-suppressed T1-weighted sequence.

B. T1-weighted sequence.

C. T2-weighted sequence.

D. Echo-planar diffusion-weighted imaging (DWI).

E. Non-echo-planar DWI.

88.3 A high postoperative recurrence rate is **MOST** associated with which of the following?

A. Extension into Prussak's space.

B. Extension into sinus tympani.

C. Ossicular erosion.

D. Canal wall down mastoidectomy.

E. Extension into the mastoid antrum.

Answers and Explanations

88.1 Correct: B. Pars flaccida cholesteatoma.

The presence of a soft tissue mass in Prussak's space, with associated erosion of the scutum or ossicles, is suggestive of a pars flaccida cholesteatoma. Pars flaccida is the smaller and superior portion of the tympanic membrane, and cholesteatomas occurring here are far more common than the pars tensa.

Other choices and discussion

A. A glomus tympanicum paraganglioma would be located on the cochlear promontory, and ossicular and bony erosion would be absent.

C. The presence of scutal and ossicular erosion in this case makes chronic otitis media a less likely diagnosis.

D. Cholesterol granuloma can occur in the middle ear with bony erosion; however, this entity does not restrict diffusion.

E. Congenital cholesteatoma may have associated ossicular erosion; however, this is typically located medial to the ossicles.

88.2 Correct: E. Non-echo-planar DWI.

Cholesteatomas are hyperintense on DWI. Non-echo-planar DWI sequences, such as HASTE or PROPELLER, are particularly useful in the imaging evaluation of cholesteatoma and best for distinguishing cholesteatoma from other entities such as granulation tissue or chronic otitis media. DWI may eliminate the need for a second-look surgery in patients who have previously undergone resection of cholesteatoma.

Other choices and discussion

D. Echo-planar DWI is the conventional form of DWI, which can demonstrate significant distortion and susceptibility artifact at the skull base and has low signal-to-noise ratio.

B, C. Cholesteatomas are typically hypointense on T1-weighted imaging (**B**) and homogeneously hyperintense on T2-weighted imaging (**C**); however, these features are not specific.

A. On postcontrast fat-suppressed T1-weighted imaging, cholesteatomas are largely nonenhancing, in contrast to inflammatory tissue; however, this feature is less specific than DWI.

88.3 Correct: B. Extension into sinus tympani.

The sinus tympani is a clinical blind spot where cholesteatoma may be hidden, and extension into the sinus tympani is associated with a high recurrence rate after surgical resection.

Other choices and discussion

D. The more extensive canal wall down mastoidectomy affords wider surgical exposure, thereby, decreasing the possibility of recurrence.

C, A, E. Ossicular erosion, (**C**) extension into Prussak's space (**A**), and extension into the mastoid antrum (**E**) are common features of cholesteatoma with no particular association with recurrence.

References

Fitzek C, Mewes T, Fitzek S, et al. Diffusion-weighted MRI of cholesteatomas of the petrous bone. *J Magn Reson Imaging.* 2002;15:636.

Schwartz KM, Lane JI, Bolster BD, et al. The utility of diffusion-weighted imaging for cholesteatoma evaluation. *AJNR Am J Neuroradiol.* 2011;32(3):430–436.

Case 89

Please refer to the following images to answer the next three questions:

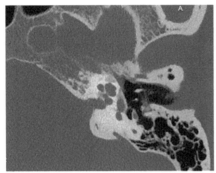

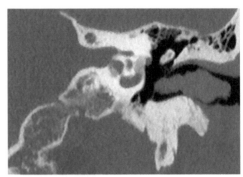

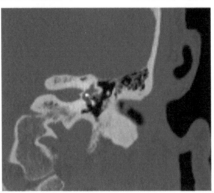

A 50-year-old healthy male presents with conductive hearing loss.

89.1 What is the **MOST** likely diagnosis?

A. Labyrinthitis ossificans.

B. Fibrous dysplasia.

C. Ossicular demineralization.

D. Osteoradionecrosis.

E. Otosclerosis.

89.2 Which is the site at which otosclerosis originates?

A. Aditus ad antrum.

B. Fissula ante fenestram.

C. Membranous labyrinth.

D. Cochlear promontory.

E. Round window niche.

89.3 What is the treatment for fenestral otosclerosis?

A. Calcium therapy.

B. Stapedectomy.

C. Cochlear implantation.

D. Sodium fluoride.

E. Bisphosphonates.

Answers and Explanations

89.1 Correct: E. Otosclerosis.

The CT images show abnormal lucency within the bony labyrinth, around the cochlea, which is compatible with the diagnosis of otosclerosis or otospongiosis. Otosclerosis is somewhat of a misnomer as CT imaging often reveals lucent (rather than sclerotic) bony changes. It most often presents bilaterally with conductive (although it can present with sensorineural or mixed) hearing loss. There are two subtypes: fenestral (which is most common and involves the oval window and stapes footplate) and retrofenestral (which involves the cochlear capsule). Retrofenestral otosclerosis usually does not occur without fenestral involvement; as such, these subtypes are considered a continuum rather than distinct entities. Both are demonstrated in the above case. Incidental note is made of cerumen in the external auditory canal.

On the axial CT image of the temporal bone, there is abnormal lucency involving the bony labyrinth, which is compatible with the diagnosis of otosclerosis. The radiodense stapes prosthesis is malpositioned with the tip posteriorly dislocated. Subluxation or dislocation is the most common cause of recurrent hearing loss following stapedectomy, occurring in 50 to 60% of these patients.

Other choices and discussion

C. While the ossicles show hypodensity consistent with demineralization (best seen on the coronal image), the main findings are in the bony labyrinth or otic capsule).

D. No prior history of skull base or nasopharyngeal radiation therapy is provided to support the diagnosis of osteoradionecrosis.

B. In fibrous dysplasia, ground-glass or sclerotic opacity rather than lucency is typical, and the inner ear is not usually involved.

A. In labyrinthitis ossificans, the membranous rather than bony labyrinth is involved, and increased rather than decreased density is expected on CT.

89.2 Correct: B. Fissula ante fenestram.

The process of otosclerosis begins at the fissula ante fenestram, which is a cleft between the inner and middle ears located at the anterior margin of the oval window.

Other choices and discussion

E. The round window is an incorrect answer as it is the oval window where otosclerosis is located.

A. The aditus ad antrum is the communication between the epitympanum of the middle ear and the mastoid cavity and is not involved with otosclerosis.

C. Otosclerosis involves the bony labyrinth; the membranous labyrinth is not directly affected.

D. Otosclerosis first occurs in the area of the fissula ante fenestram (fenestral), and then progresses to involve the cochlear promontory, vestibule, and otic capsule (retrofenestral).

89.3 Correct: B. Stapedectomy.

Stapedectomy with prosthesis placement is the treatment of choice for fenestral otosclerosis.

Other choices and discussion

A, E. Calcium therapy (**A**) and bisphosphonates (**E**) are not used in the treatment of otosclerosis.

D. Sodium fluoride therapy is used in cases of cochlear otosclerosis.

C. Cochlear implantation can be offered in cases of profound mixed hearing loss, resulting from concurrent fenestral and cochlear otosclerosis; however, this is not typical.

References

Purohit B, Hermans R, Op de beeck K. Imaging in otosclerosis: A pictorial review. Insights Imaging. 2014;5(2): 245–252.

Stone JA, Mukherji SK, Jewett BS, et al. CT Evaluation of Prosthetic Ossicular Reconstruction: What the Otologist Needs to Know. Radiographics. 2000;20(3): 593–605.

Case 90

Please refer to the following images to answer the next three questions:

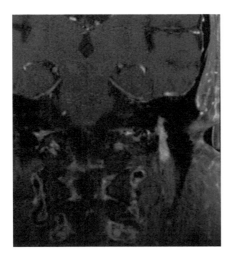

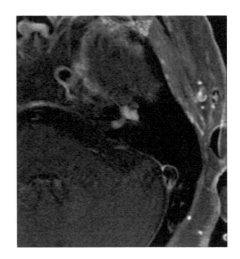

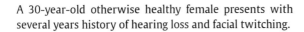

A 30-year-old otherwise healthy female presents with several years history of hearing loss and facial twitching.

90.1 What is the **MOST** likely diagnosis?

A. Glomus jugulare.

B. Bell's palsy.

C. Facial nerve schwannoma.

D. Facial nerve hemangioma.

E. Perineural spread of malignancy.

90.2 What is the **MOST** common location of a facial nerve schwannoma?

A. Geniculate ganglion.

B. Cerebellopontine angle/internal auditory canal.

C. Mastoid air cells.

D. Parotid gland.

E. Middle ear cavity.

90.3 A facial nerve tumor involving which branch or segment of the facial nerve projects into the middle cranial fossa?

A. Temporal branch.

B. Chorda tympani.

C. Tympanic segment.

D. Mastoid segment.

E. Greater superficial petrosal nerve.

Answers and Explanations

90.1 Correct: C. Facial nerve schwannoma.

On the axial and coronal postcontrast fat-suppressed MR images, note the tubular, homogeneously enhancing, and smoothly marginated mass which follows the course of the facial nerve in the left temporal bone. These imaging features are most consistent with a facial nerve schwannoma.

Other choices and discussion

A. The marginated mass is not located in the jugular foramen and, therefore, does not represent a glomus jugulare.
B, D. Bell's palsy (**B**) and facial nerve hemangioma (**C**) would be expected to have a more acute clinical presentation.
E. Perineural spread of malignancy is less likely because of the absence of known malignancy in this otherwise healthy patient.

90.2 Correct: A. Geniculate ganglion.

The geniculate ganglion fossa is the most common location of a facial nerve schwannoma, and schwannomas located here can extend to the tympanic or labyrinthine segments. A typical facial nerve schwannoma involves more than one segment of the facial nerve.

Other choices and discussion

B–E. Facial nerve schwannomas can occur in the cerebellopontine angle/internal auditory canal (**B**), middle ear cavity (**E**), mastoid air cells (**C**), and parotid gland (**D**); however, these locations are less commonly involved.

90.3 Correct: E. Greater superficial petrosal nerve.

The greater superficial petrosal nerve projects anteromedially and cephalad from the geniculate fossa into the middle cranial fossa. A facial nerve schwannoma involving the greater superficial petrosal nerve should, therefore, be considered in the case of an ovoid middle cranial fossa mass.

Other choices and discussion

A. A schwannoma involving the temporal branch would be extracranial in location.
B–D. A schwannoma involving the chorda tympani (**B**), tympanic segment (**C**), and mastoid segment (**D**) would be intratemporal in location.

References

Mundada P, Purohit BS, Kumar TS, et al. Imaging of facial nerve schwannomas: diagnostic pearls and potential pitfalls. Diagn Interv Radiol. 2016;22(1):40–46.

Wiggins RH 3rd, Harnsberger HR, Salzman KL, et al. The many faces of facial nerve schwannoma. AJNR Am J Neuroradiol. 27(3):694-699, 2006

Case 91

Please refer to the following images to answer the next three questions:

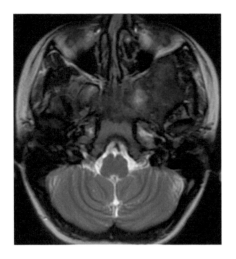

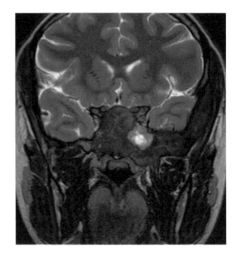

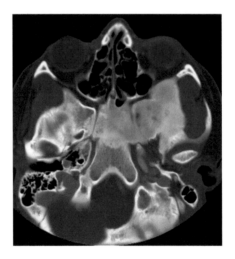

A 24-year-old female with daily headache.

91.1 What is the **MOST** likely diagnosis?

A. Chondrosarcoma.
B. Fibrous dysplasia.
C. Chordoma.
D. Ossifying fibroma.
E. Paget's disease.

91.2 What is the **BEST** next step in management?

A. Positron emission tomography (PET)/CT scan.
B. Consultation with skull base surgeon for biopsy.
C. CT head.
D. Follow-up MRI in 6 months.
E. Bone scan.

91.3 What is the typical pattern of uptake on a nuclear medicine bone scan for this diagnosis?

A. Decreased in perfusion phase.
B. Decreased in blood pool phase.
C. Decreased unless an active lesion.
D. Variable.
E. Increased in perfusion phase and decreased in delayed phase.

Answers and Explanations

91.1   Correct: B. Fibrous dysplasia.

On the axial and coronal T2-weighted MR images, note the expansile appearance of the sphenoid bone and left temporal calvarium which is predominantly hypointense in signal on T2-weighted imaging. On the noncontrast axial CT image, there is corresponding ground-glass opacity in this region which makes fibrous dysplasia the most likely diagnosis. The enhancement pattern of fibrous dysplasia is variable. A small internal focus of hyperintense signal is compatible with cystic change.

Other choices and discussion

A, C. Chondrosarcoma (**A**) and chordoma (**C**), in contrast, are expected to demonstrate predominantly hyperintense signal on T2-weighted imaging.
D. Ossifying fibroma is also an expansile mass, but the expansion is concentric and more spherical and tumor-like. The expansion demonstrated in these images maintains the general shape of the involved bone, which is typical of fibrous dysplasia.
E. The appearance of Paget's disease is one of mixed lysis and sclerosis on CT and heterogeneous signal on MRI, which is inconsistent with the appearance seen here. In addition, Paget's disease is less likely to occur in a younger female patient.

91.2   Correct: C. CT head.

The MRI appearance of fibrous dysplasia is highly variable and can mimic neoplasm or other aggressive processes. Therefore, CT scan of head should be obtained and evaluated in bone windows to assess for the typical ground glass opacity of fibrous dysplasia and better define the extent of involvement. In this case, CT showed ground-glass opacity, rendering a diagnosis of fibrous dysplasia, and no intervention was undertaken. In the skull base, this condition can lead to cranial nerve palsy, facial pain, or headache.

Other choices and discussion

A. PET/CT scan can incidentally demonstrate variable uptake in fibrous dysplasia; however, this is not needed to establish the diagnosis.
E. Bone scan can be used to define the extent of lesions in polyostotic fibrous dysplasia; however, in this case, the diagnosis needs to be established first with CT.
B. Consultation with a skull base surgeon for biopsy is not needed, given the natural history and prognosis of fibrous dysplasia.
D. No follow-up MR imaging is indicated unless there is a change of symptoms or increased pain which may indicate malignant transformation.

91.3   Correct: D. Variable.

There is variable and nonspecific 99m-Tc MDP radionuclide uptake on nuclear medicine bone scan.

Other choices and discussion

A–C, E. Most instances of fibrous dyplasia show increased uptake, most markedly in the delayed phase but also in the early perfusion phase. However other foci, especially when cystic, demonstrate no increased tracer uptake. The findings on bone scan should always be correlated with radiographs or CT and are particularly useful in mapping the lesions in polyostotic fibrous dysplasia.

References

Kransdorf MJ, Moser RP, Gilkey FW. Fibrous dysplasia. *Radiographics*. 1990;10:519–537.

Jee WH, Choi KH, Choe BY, et al. Fibrous dysplasia: MR imaging characteristics with radiopathologic correlation. *AJR Am J Roentgenol*. 1996;167(6):1523–1527.

Zhibin Y, Quanyong L, Libo C, et al. The role of radionuclide bone scintigraphy in fibrous dysplasia of bone. *Clin Nucl Med*. 2004;29(3):177–180.

Case 92

Please refer to the following images to answer the next three questions:

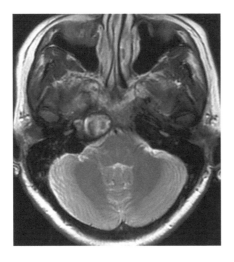
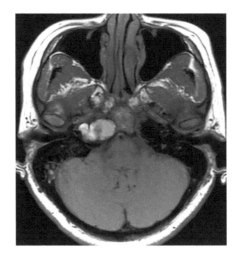

A 35-year-old female presents with dizziness.

92.1 What is the **MOST** likely diagnosis?

A. Asymmetric pneumatization of the petrous apex.

B. Cholesteatoma.

C. Cholesterol granuloma.

D. Petrous apicitis.

E. Trapped fluid in petrous apex.

92.2 Which of the following structures immediately borders the petrous apex?

A. Internal auditory canal.

B. Pterygopalatine fossa.

C. Cavernous internal carotid artery.

D. Inferior orbital fissure.

E. Facial recess.

92.3 Which of the following is characteristic of the imaging appearance of cholesterol granuloma?

A. Restricted diffusion.

B. True enhancement.

C. Permeative bony margins.

D. Hypointensity on T2-weighted sequence.

E. High signal on T1-weighted imaging.

Answers and Explanations

92.1   Correct: C. Cholesterol granuloma.

On the T1-weighted image, there is an expansile and lobulated lesion in the right petrous apex with intrinsic hyperintense signal. On the T2-weighted image, the lesion has a hypointense rim reflecting hemosiderin deposition. The imaging findings are consistent with a cholesterol granuloma, the most common primary lesion of the petrous apex.

Other choices and discussion

B, D. Congenital cholesteatoma (**B**) occurring in the petrous apex and petrous apicitis (**D**) would be expected to show low-to-intermediate signal intensity on T1-weighted imaging.
E, A. Trapped fluid in the petrous apex (**E**) or marrow due to asymmetric pneumatization (**A**) can appear similar to a cholesterol granuloma in terms of MRI signal intensity; however, there is no associated expansion or destruction of the petrous apex air cells with these entities.

92.2   Correct: C. Cavernous internal carotid artery.

The petrous apex has critical relationships with several adjacent structures in the skull base including cranial nerves. In fact, the clinical presentation of a cholesterol granuloma can often be attributable to the invasion of adjacent structures, and temporal bone CT is useful for delineating bony erosion and subsequent involvement of these critical structures.

Other choices and discussion

A. The petrous apex is anteromedial to the internal auditory canal. The vertical and horizontal petrous segments of the internal carotid artery immediately border the petrous apex; however, the cavernous segment does not.

E. The facial recess is located along the posterior wall of the middle ear cavity and not immediately adjacent to the petrous apex.
B, D. The pterygopalatine fossa (**B**) and the inferior orbital fissure (**D**) are both located more anteriorly within the skull base.

92.3   Correct: E. High signal on T1-weighted imaging.

Classic cholesterol granulomas have high signal on T1-weighted imaging, related to cholesterol crystals and/or blood products.

Other choices and discussion

B. There is intrinsic hyperintensity on T1-weighted imaging but no true enhancement in a cholesterol granuloma.
D. A cholesterol granuloma characteristically appears hyperintense on T2-weighted imaging, not hypointense.
A. There is no restricted diffusion associated with a cholesterol granuloma; presence of restricted diffusion in the petrous apex could instead indicate cholesteatoma or petrous apicitis complicated by abscess.
C. Sharp, not permeative, bony margins on CT are typical of a petrous apex cholesterol granuloma. Larger lesions can demonstrate areas of bony dehiscence, and these should be reported to the surgeon.

References

Chapman PR, Shah R, Curé JK, et al. Petrous Apex Lesions: Pictorial Review. *AJR Am J Roentgenol.* 2011;196(3 Suppl): WS26–WS37.

Juliano AF, Ginat DT, Moonis G. Imaging Review of the Temporal Bone: Part I. Anatomy and Inflammatory and Neoplastic Processes. *Radiology.* 2013;269(1):17–33.

Case 93

Please refer to the following images to answer the next three questions:

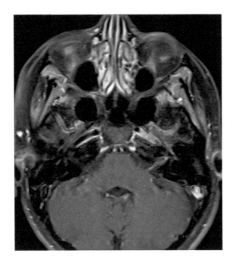 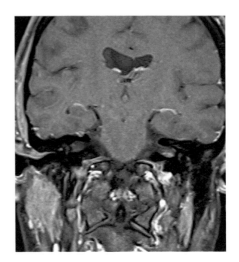

A 50-year-old previously healthy female presents with an eight-day history of left facial weakness, mild left hearing loss, and imbalance.

93.1 Which cranial nerves demonstrate abnormal enhancement?

A. Cranial nerve VII, left.

B. Cranial nerve VII, bilateral.

C. Cranial nerves VII and VIII, left.

D. Cranial nerves VII and VIII, bilateral.

E. Cochlear and vestibular nerves, left.

93.2 What is the **MOST** likely diagnosis?

A. Bell's palsy.

B. Ramsay Hunt syndrome.

C. Perineural spread.

D. Facial nerve schwannoma.

E. Vestibular schwannoma.

93.3 Which segment or branch of the facial nerve does not normally enhance in the temporal bone?

A. Canalicular IAC segment.

B. Greater superficial petrosal nerve.

C. Geniculate ganglion.

D. Tympanic segment.

E. Mastoid.

Answers and Explanations

93.1 Correct: C. Cranial nerves VII and VIII, left.

On the axial postcontrast fat-suppressed image, there is abnormal linear enhancement in both the anterior and posterior aspects of the left internal auditory canal, corresponding to the left facial (CN VII) and superior vestibular (CN VIII) nerves, respectively. On the coronal postcontrast fat-suppressed image, there is also abnormal enhancement, corresponding to the mastoid segment of the left facial nerve. In the internal auditory canal, the facial nerve is anterior and superior, and the cochlear nerve is anterior and inferior ("seven up, coke down"). The superior and inferior vestibular nerves are posterior in location.

Other choices and discussion
A, B, D, E. These answer choices are incorrect because the only enhancing nerves that are shown in the images are cranial nerves VII and VIII on the left.

93.2 Correct: B. Ramsay Hunt syndrome.

The imaging findings of abnormal enhancement of the facial and vestibulocochlear nerves and membranous labyrinth are compatible with Ramsay Hunt syndrome, also known as herpes zoster oticus. On physical examination, this patient demonstrated erythematous crusted vesicles in the external ear, which are characteristic of this diagnosis. In Ramsay Hunt syndrome, facial nerve enhancement most prominently involves the segments in the fundus of the internal auditory canal (IAC) and fallopian canal (labyrinthine segment).

Other choices and discussion
A. Bell's palsy may also demonstrate facial nerve (CN VII) enhancement; however, there is usually no enhancement of the vestibulocochlear nerve (CN VIII) or membranous labyrinth.

C. Perineural spread is less likely in the absence of a known primary malignancy, such as squamous cell carcinoma of the face or scalp or parotid malignancy.
D. Facial nerve schwannoma is incorrect because the vestibulocochlear nerve is also involved.
E. Similarly, vestibular schwannoma is also incorrect because the facial nerve also enhances abnormally.

93.3 Correct: A. Canalicular IAC segment.

The cisternal, canalicular, and labyrinthine segments of the facial nerve do not normally enhance due to lack of a perineural vascular plexus.

Other choices and discussion
B–D. The normal circumneural arteriovenous plexus, which feeds the facial nerve in the facial canal, can be responsible for mild enhancement of the geniculate ganglion, greater superficial petrosal nerve, and proximal tympanic segment.
E. The mastoid segment can also show enhancement due to high capillary density. In contrast, the cisternal and canalicular segments do not normally enhance due to lack of this plexus.

References

Lustig LR, Niparko JK. Chapter 70. Disorders of the Facial Nerve. In: Lalwani AK. eds. CURRENT Diagnosis & Treatment in Otolaryngology—Head & Neck Surgery, 3e, New York, NY: McGraw-Hill; 2012.

Sartoretti-Schefer S, Kollias S, Valavanis A. Ramsay Hunt syndrome associated with brain stem enhancement. *AJNR Am J Neuroradiol.* 1999;20:278–280.

Case 94

Please refer to the following images to answer the next three questions:

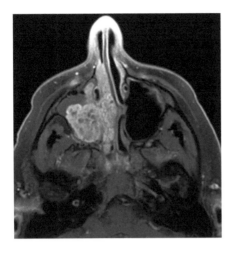 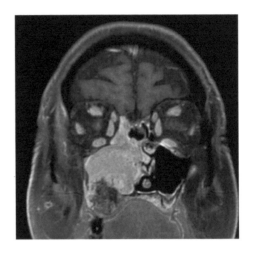

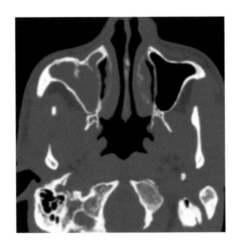

A 44-year-old female presents with long-standing right nasal airway obstruction.

94.1 What is the **MOST** likely diagnosis?

A. Sinonasal polyposis.

B. Antrochoanal polyp.

C. Juvenile nasopharyngeal angiofibroma.

D. Sinonasal adenocarcinoma.

E. Inverted papilloma.

94.2 What is the associated malignancy with this diagnosis?

A. Adenocarcinoma.

B. Melanoma.

C. Squamous cell carcinoma.

D. Esthesioneuroblastoma.

E. Sinonasal undifferentiated carcinoma.

94.3 Which virus is suspected in the pathogenesis of inverted papilloma?

A. Human immunodeficiency virus (HIV).

B. Human herpes virus (HHV).

C. Varicella zoster virus (VZV).

D. Human papilloma virus (HPV).

E. EpsteinBarr virus (EBV).

Answers and Explanations

94.1   Correct: E. Inverted papilloma.

On the axial and coronal postcontrast fat-suppressed MR images, note the convoluted cerebriform pattern of contrast enhancement within the tumor, which is characteristic of inverted papilloma. On the axial noncontrast CT in a different patient, the focal hyperostosis along the anterior wall of the right maxillary sinus indicates a bony strut that is the site of attachment for the tumor. Complete resection of the osseous strut decreases the rate of recurrence and, accordingly, the site of attachment to the nasal cavity or sinus wall should be reported to the surgeon.

Other choices and discussion

A, B. Sinonasal polyposis (**A**) and antrochoanal polyp (**B**) typically demonstrate peripheral enhancement only, making these choices less likely.
C. Juvenile nasopharyngeal angiofibroma is unlikely in a middle-aged female; in addition, this entity would be expected to be centered in the posterior nasal cavity.
D. Sinonasal adenocarcinoma is less likely due to its predilection for the ethmoid sinus.

94.2   Correct: C. Squamous cell carcinoma.

Inverted papilloma may harbor or degenerate into squamous cell carcinoma (SCC) in an estimated 5 to 15% of patients. Synchronous-associated SCC is more common than metachronous SCC. On the coronal postcontrast fat-suppressed MR images, note the loss of convoluted cerebriform pattern of enhancement inferiorly in the alveolar recess of the maxillary sinus, which was confirmed to be a focus of synchronous SCC within a background of inverted papilloma.

Other choices and discussion

A. Sinonasal adenocarcinoma can appear similar to SCC on imaging; however, adenocarcinoma has a predilection for the ethmoid cavity.

B. Melanoma has a predilection for the nasal cavity and can sometimes show increased T1 signal, which is related to melanin content or hemorrhage.
D. Esthesioneuroblastoma has a predilection for the superior nasal cavity and frequently demonstrates transcranial extension.
E. The imaging appearance of sinonasal undifferentiated carcinoma overlaps with that of SCC; however, there is no particular association with inverted papilloma.

94.3   Correct: D. Human papilloma virus (HPV).

Although the pathogenesis of inverted papilloma remains uncertain, there is increasing evidence of an association with HPV, which already has a more established role in other head and neck neoplasms. Higher rates of malignancy and recurrence are encountered in inverted papillomas if HPV is present in the pathology specimen. Other proposed risk factors for inverted papilloma include occupational exposure to aerosols and other inhaled noxious agents.

Other choices and discussion

E. Nasopharyngeal carcinoma has a strong association with EBV.
B. The multicentric form of Castleman disease is associated with HHV.
A. HIV is associated with malignancies such as lymphoma and Kaposi's sarcoma.
C. VZV is associated with Ramsay Hunt syndrome.

References

Jeon TY, Kim HJ, Chung SK, et al. Sinonasal Inverted Papilloma: Value of Convoluted Cerebriform Pattern on MR Imaging. *AJNR Am J Neuroradiol.* 2008;29(8):1556–1560.

Lee DK, Chung SK, Dhong HJ, et al. Focal Hyperostosis on CT of Sinonasal Inverted Papilloma as a Predictor of Tumor Origin. *AJNR Am J Neuroradiol.* 2007;28(4):618–621.

Case 95

Please refer to the following images to answer the next three questions:

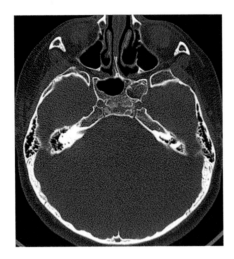
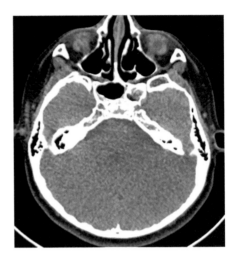

A 9-year-old female with sinusitis.

95.1 What is the **MOST** likely diagnosis?

A. Arrested pneumatization of the sphenoid sinus.

B. Chondrosarcoma.

C. Ossifying fibroma.

D. Chordoma.

E. Fibrous dysplasia.

95.2 What is the **BEST** next step in management?

A. No further steps are necessary.

B. Biopsy.

C. Contrast-enhanced CT.

D. Further evaluation with MRI.

E. Bone scan.

95.3 Which of the following structures immediately borders the sphenoid sinus?

A. Optic nerve.

B. Cribriform plate.

C. Sphenotemporal suture.

D. Foramen ovale.

E. Foramen spinosum.

Answers and Explanations

95.1 Correct: A. Arrested pneumatization of the sphenoid sinus.

On the axial CT images in bone and soft tissue windows, there is a nonexpansile fat density lesion with well-circumscribed sclerotic borders in the left basisphenoid. The immediately adjacent vidian canal is preserved. This appearance is most compatible with arrested pneumatization, a benign developmental variant which is usually associated with the sphenoid sinus. Internal calcifications can also be seen with this entity.

Other choices and discussion
B, D. Chondrosarcoma (**B**) and chordoma (**D**) are expansile destructive lesions without internal fat content.
C. Although an ossifying fibroma would be circumscribed, as seen in this case, it would be expected to appear as an expansile lesion that is usually located in the mandible, sinonasal region, and orbits rather than the skull base.
E. This lesion is also not consistent with fibrous dysplasia which commonly demonstrates ground-glass opacity; in addition, fibrous dysplasia is usually expansile and narrows the adjacent neural foramina.

95.2 Correct: A. No further steps are necessary.

Arrested pneumatization is a "do NOT touch" lesion of the skull base and incidentally encountered on many CT and MRI studies. Arrested pneumatization can be confidently diagnosed if the lesion in question is nonexpansile with a well-circumscribed sclerotic border, has fatty contents, and occurs in a site of normal or accessory pneumatization. Internal calcifications are usually present, and adjacent neural and vascular foramina are preserved.

Other choices and discussion
B. Biopsy is not indicated.
D. MRI can be obtained to confirm the fatty nature of the lesion but is usually not necessary in cases where the imaging appearance is classic.
C, E. Contrast-enhanced CT (**C**) and bone scan (**E**) and bone scan are also not necessary in this case.

95.3 Correct: A. Optic nerve.

The optic nerve is superior to the sphenoid sinus and medial to the anterior clinoid process.

Other choices and discussion
B. The cribriform plate is part of the ethmoid bone within the anterior skull base and not along the border of the sphenoid sinus.
C. The sphenotemporal suture is located within the lateral orbital rim and does not border the sphenoid sinus.
D, E. Foramen ovale (**D**) and foramen spinosum (**E**) are located in the greater wing of the sphenoid and not immediately adjacent to the sphenoid sinus.

References

Kuntzler S, Jankowski R. Arrested pneumatization: witness of paranasal sinuses development? *Eur Ann Otorhinolaryngol Head Neck Dis.* 2014;131(3):167–170.

Welker KM, DeLone DR, Lane JI, et al. Arrested pneumatization of the skull base: imaging characteristics. *AJR Am J Roentgenol.* 2008;190(6):1691–1696.

Case 96

Challenge

Please refer to the following images to answer the next three questions:

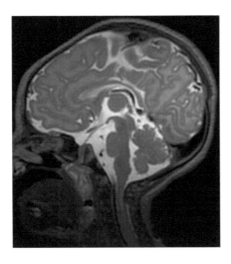

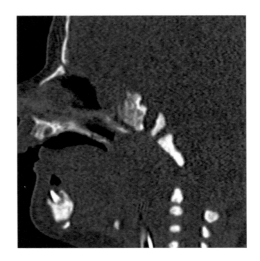

An 8-day-old girl presents with nasopharyngeal mass.

96.1   What is the **MOST** likely diagnosis?

A. Teratoma.

B. Ectopic thyroid tissue.

C. Invasive pituitary adenoma.

D. Persistent sphenooccipital synchondrosis.

E. Persistent craniopharyngeal canal.

96.2   What is the leading hypothesis regarding the origin of this lesion?

A. Arrested development of the sphenoid sinus.

B. Remnant of a vascular channel.

C. Failure of Rathke pouch to close.

D. Duplication of the sphenooccipital synchondrosis.

E. Overgrowth of a pituitary neoplasm.

96.3   Which of the following is **TRUE** of this diagnosis?

A. Surgery reduces the risk of cerebrospinal fluid (CSF) leak.

B. Ectopic thyroid gland is often also present.

C. Classification of this diagnosis into three types is based on the age of the patient.

D. Small incidental canals do not require surgery.

E. Hypotelorism is associated with this entity.

Answers and Explanations

96.1 Correct: E. Persistent craniopharyngeal canal.

On the sagittal T2-weighted MR image and sagittal non-contrast CT image in the bone window, a prominent tract is seen extending anteroinferiorly from the pituitary fossa to the nasopharynx through which the pituitary gland herniates inferiorly. Findings are consistent with a large dilated persistent craniopharyngeal canal.

Other choices and discussion
C. The pituitary gland is present within the herniated tissue; however, there is no evidence of invasive pituitary adenoma.
D. The sphenoccipital synchondrosis is normally open at this age and positioned anteroinferiorly to the persistent craniopharyngeal canal.
A, B. Teratoma (**A**) and ectopic thyroid tissue (**B**) are not present.

96.2 Correct: C. Failure of Rathke pouch to close.

The adenohypophyseal (Rathke) stalk normally obliterates by the 12th week of gestation. The abnormal persistence of this tract is thought to be responsible for the entity of the persistent craniopharyngeal canal.

Other choices and discussion
B. Previously, the prevailing theory was that the persistent craniopharyngeal canal is the remnant of a vascular channel; however, existing evidence does not support this explanation.
D, E, A. Duplication of the sphenooccipital synchondrosis (**D**), overgrowth of a pituitary neoplasm (**E**), and arrested development of the sphenoid sinus (**A**) are not thought to be responsible for the finding of persistent craniopharyngeal canal.

96.3 Correct: D. Small incidental canals do not require surgery.

Small incidental canals are "don't touch" lesions which do not require surgery.

Other choices and discussion
A. Surgery increases, rather than decreases, the risk of CSF leak, especially when cephaloceles are present.
B. Ectopic thyroid gland has no association with this entity; however, ectopic pituitary gland can be present within the nasopharynx in the case of large craniopharyngeal canals.
C. Classification of this diagnosis is based on the size of the canal and content (small, medium, or large); classification does not depend on the age of the patient.
E. Hypertelorism, not hypotelorism, in combination with a nasopharyngeal mass should prompt further workup, with imaging of the skull base to evaluate for this entity.

References

Abele TA, Salzman KL, Harnsberger HR, et al. Craniopharyngeal canal and its spectrum of pathology. *AJNR Am J Neuroradiol.* 2014;35:772–777.

Kaushik C, Ramakrishnaiah R, Angtuaco EJ. Ectopic pituitary adenoma in persistent craniopharyngeal canal: case report and literature review. *J Comput Assist Tomogr.* 2010;34:612–614.

Case 97

Challenge

Please refer to the following images to answer the next three questions:

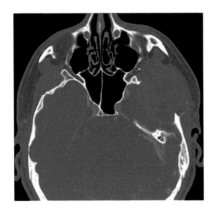
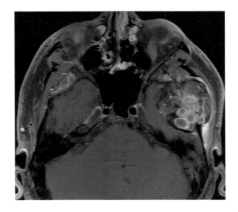
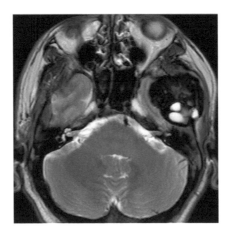

A 38-year-old otherwise healthy female presents with left facial pain and swelling.

97.1 What is the **MOST** likely diagnosis?

A. Chordoma.

B. Giant cell tumor (GCT).

C. Fibrous dysplasia.

D. Chondrosarcoma.

E. Metastasis.

97.2 Which of the following locations is **MOST** common for this diagnosis?

A. Frontal bone.

B. Sphenoid bone.

C. Temporal bone.

D. Parietal bone.

E. Occipital bone.

97.3 Which is a known complication of GCT?

A. Accelerated growth during pregnancy.

B. Bone infarct.

C. Osteonecrosis.

D. Malignant degeneration to squamous cell carcinoma.

E. Aneurysmal bone cyst.

Answers and Explanations

97.1 Correct: B. Giant cell tumor (GCT).

The axial T1-weighted fat-suppressed postcontrast and T2-weighted images show a well-circumscribed, expansile, and heterogeneously enhancing intraosseous mass centered in the squamous portion of the left temporal bone. The appearance and location are characteristic of giant cell tumor. Markedly hypointense internal signal on T2-weighted imaging is typical of GCT in the temporal bone and reflects extensive hemosiderin deposition or calcification. There is medial extension into the middle cranial fossa with mass effect on the left temporal lobe, which is characteristic for this lesion and location.

Other choices and discussion

A, D. Chordoma (**A**) and chondrosarcoma (**D**) reliably demonstrate signal hyperintensity on T2-weighted imaging, which is not present in this case.
C. Fibrous dysplasia is expected in patients under the age of 30 and there is usually less enhancement than seen with GCT.
E. Metastasis is unlikely in a young and otherwise healthy patient.

97.2 Correct: B. Sphenoid bone.

The calvarium is an uncommon location of GCT and only accounts for 2% of cases. However, of the calvarial locations of GCT, the sphenoid bone is the most common.

Other choices and discussion

C. Following the sphenoid bone, the temporal bone is the second most common location.

A, D, E. The frontal bone (**A**), parietal bone (**D**), and occipital bone (**E**) are exceedingly rare locations for GCTs.

97.3 Correct: E. Aneurysmal bone cyst.

An aneurysmal bone cyst can arise secondarily within a GCT, and the presence of an aneurysmal bone cyst is suggested by fluidfluid levels within the GCT.

Other choices and discussion

A. Accelerated growth during pregnancy is associated with giant cell reparative granuloma, but not GCT.
B, C. Bone infarct (**B**) and osteonecrosis (**C**) have no association with GCT.
D. Malignant degeneration to sarcoma, not squamous cell carcinoma, is a potential complication of GCT.

References

Chakarun CJ, Forrester DM, Gottsegen CJ, et al. Giant cell tumor of bone: review, mimics, and new developments in treatment. *Radiographics*. 2013;33(1):197–211.

Kashiwagi N, Hirabuki N, Andou K, et al. MRI and CT findings of the giant cell tumors of the skull; five cases and a review of the literature. *Eur J Radiol*. 2006;58(3):435–443.

Kunimatsu A, Kunimatsu N. Skull base tumors and tumor-like lesions: a pictorial review. *Pol J Radiol*. 2017;82:398–409.

Case 98

Challenge

Please refer to the following images to answer the next three questions:

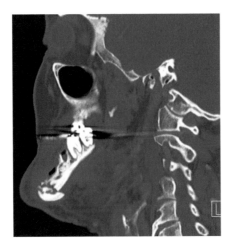
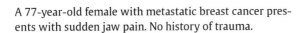
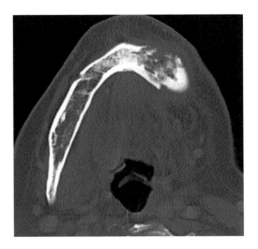

A 77-year-old female with metastatic breast cancer presents with sudden jaw pain. No history of trauma.

98.1 What is the **MOST** likely diagnosis?

A. Paget's disease.

B. Medication-related osteonecrosis of the jaw.

C. Osseous metastasis.

D. Osteoradionecrosis.

E. Langerhans histiocytosis.

98.2 What is the complication demonstrated here?

A. Pathologic fracture.

B. Abscess.

C. Perineural tumor spread.

D. Maxillary sinusitis.

E. Giant cell tumor.

98.3 Which of the following is **TRUE** of the diagnosis?

A. The diagnosis does not occur in the maxilla.

B. Biopsy is often needed to confirm the diagnosis.

C. Hyperbaric oxygen therapy is an effective treatment.

D. Increased uptake on a nuclear medicine bone scan is present in the majority of cases.

E. Discontinuation of the offending medication can reverse the bone destruction.

Answers and Explanations

98.1 Correct: B. Medication-related osteonecrosis of the jaw.

The sagittal and axial noncontrast CT images in bone window demonstrate ill-defined areas of lucency and permeative cortical erosion in the left parasymphyseal mandible. There is also a likely sequestrum demonstrated on the sagittal image. On further query, the patient reported a 10-year history of bisphosphonate medication use which had been prescribed for bone metastases secondary to breast cancer. Overall, the findings in conjunction with the initially unknown clinical history of bisphosphonate use are compatible with advanced bisphosphonate-related osteonecrosis of the jaw. Focal medullary sclerosis is an early imaging finding of osteonecrosis. Periosteal reaction and bony sequestrum are imaging features of advanced stages of osteonecrosis. Persistent alveolar socket after tooth extraction (not seen here) is also highly characteristic of osteonecrosis of the jaw.

Other choices and discussion

A. Paget's disease is unlikely because the imaging findings in Paget's are of diffuse expansion of the entire jaw, with internal ground-glass and cortical thickening, rather than the focal lytic changes seen in this case.

C. Osseous metastasis is possible, although less likely in the absence of an associated soft tissue mass.

D. History of oral cavity or oropharynx squamous cell carcinoma and treatment with radiation therapy to the mandible would be expected for osteoradionecrosis, which can have a similar appearance; however, there is no such history in the above case.

E. Langerhans histiocytosis is more typical in a young patient with a well-circumscribed lytic lesion and a "beveled edge" appearance.

98.2 Correct: A. Pathologic fracture.

The sagittal image best shows the pathologic fracture, which has complicated this case of osteonecrosis of the jaw, and likely explains the sudden onset of jaw pain in this patient. Pathologic fracture is a common complication which was found in half of the patients in one study.

Other choices and discussion

B. Although soft tissue swelling can be present when the osteonecrosis is advanced or when complication by infection or a pathologic fracture has occurred, there is no rim-enhancing fluid collection in this case to suggest the presence of an abscess.

C. There is likely involvement of osteonecrosis of the left inferior alveolar canal, near the mental foramen, as seen on the axial image; however, no malignant involvement to support the presence of perineural tumor spread is present.

D. The partially visualized maxillary sinus on the sagittal image is clear; however, maxillary sinusitis can be associated with cases of osteonecrosis of the maxilla, rather than of the mandible.

E. Giant cell tumor transformation is a complication of Paget's disease and not of osteonecrosis of the jaw.

98.3 Correct: D. Increased uptake on a nuclear medicine bone scan is present in the majority of cases.

Increased uptake on bone scan is seen in 60 to 90% of cases of osteonecrosis of the jaw, although decreased uptake can be seen in early stages of disease.

Other choices and discussion

A. The diagnosis of bisphosphonate-related osteonecrosis does occur in the maxilla, but much less commonly than in the mandible.

B. Biopsy can worsen osteonecrosis of the jaw and should be avoided; the diagnosis should be made clinically on the basis of bone exposure present for at least 8 weeks in a patient who has received bisphosphonate therapy but not radiation.

C. Hyperbaric oxygen therapy as a treatment for bisphosphonate-related osteonecrosis is controversial and has not been shown to be particularly effective.

E. Although discontinuation of the bisphosphonate therapy is indicated when there is evidence of osteonecrosis, no therapy has been shown to reverse the bone necrosis.

References

Morag Y, Morag-Hezroni M, Jamadar DA, et al. Bisphosphonate-related osteonecrosis of the jaw: a pictorial review. *Radiographics.* 2009;29(7):1971–1984.

Ruggiero SL, Mehotra B, Rosenberg TJ, et al. Osteonecrosis of the jaws associated with the use of bisphosphonates: a review of 63 cases. *J Oral Maxillofac Surg.* 2004;62:527–534.

Challenge

Please refer to the following images to answer the next three questions:

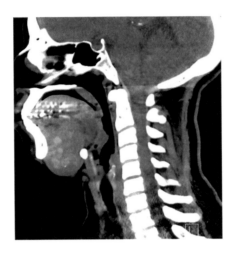

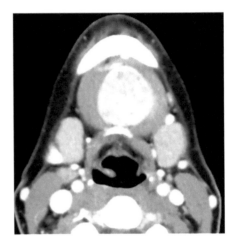

A 34-year-old female with large submental mass.

99.1   What is the **MOST** likely diagnosis?

A. Sialolithiasis.

B. Ranula.

C. Dermoid.

D. Thyroglossal duct cyst.

E. Ectopic thyroid.

99.2   Which of the following scans can **BEST** confirm the diagnosis?

A. Ultrasound.

B. Radioiodine scan.

C. Positron emission tomography (PET)/CT scan.

D. Octreotide scan.

E. MRI.

99.3   What is the **MOST** common location for this diagnosis?

A. Submandibular gland.

B. Base of tongue.

C. Sublingual space.

D. Mediastinum.

E. Root of tongue.

Answers and Explanations

99.1   Correct: E. Ectopic thyroid.

On the sagittal noncontrast CT image of the neck, a large rounded mass in the floor of the mouth, with intrinsic hyperdensity characteristic of thyroidal tissue, is shown. On the axial postcontrast CT image, the mass demonstrates avid and diffuse enhancement which is also typical of thyroidal tissue. Absence of normal thyroid gland in its typical location can also be noted in the sagittal image. Findings are consistent with ectopic lingual thyroid.

Other choices and discussion

D. The major differential consideration for a midline neck mass is a thyroglossal duct cyst; however, a thyroglossal duct cyst appears as a simple and noncalcified cyst on imaging rather than an enhancing solid mass.
A. Although poorly calcified sialoliths can show intrinsic hyperdensity on noncontrast CT, the avid enhancement is not compatible with this diagnosis.
B. Although ranulas do occur in the sublingual space, the images presented here do not demonstrate the unilateral cystic appearance or morphology of a ranula.
C. Similarly, although dermoids do present in a lingual location, the typical cystic appearance with fatty or fluid contents of a dermoid is not seen here.

99.2   Correct: B. Radioiodine scan.

Radioiodine I-123 uptake scan can be helpful in confirming the diagnosis of ectopic thyroid gland and can also aid in demonstrating the presence of functioning thyroid tissue in the typical thyroid location and elsewhere.

Other choices and discussion
A, C, E. The findings on ultrasound, PET/CT scan, and MRI are helpful in demonstrating similar imaging features of normal thyroid gland, but are not as specific with regard to confirming the diagnosis as the nuclear medicine radioiodine uptake scan.
D. Octreotide scans are used in the evaluation of neuroendocrine tumors and play no role in the workup of suspected ectopic thyroid gland.

99.3   Correct: B. Base of tongue.

The most common location of ectopic thyroid gland is the base of the tongue.

Other choices and discussion
C, E. Less common locations are the sublingual space and root of the tongue.
A. Even less common is the submandibular gland.
D. The mediastinum is a classic location for ectopic parathyroid, not thyroid, tissue.

References

Damiano A, Glickman AB, Rubin JS, et al. Ectopic thyroid tissue presenting as a midline neck mass. *Int J Pediatr Otorhinolaryngol.* 1996; 34(1–2):141–148.

Zander DA, Smoker WR: Imaging of ectopic thyroid tissue and thyroglossal duct cysts. *Radiographics.* 2014;34(1):37–50.

Case 100

Challenge

Please refer to the following images to answer the next three questions:

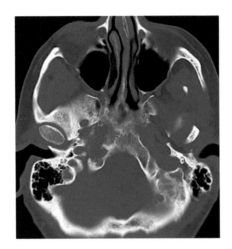

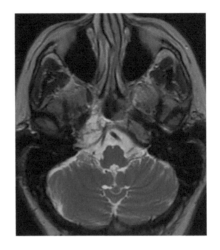

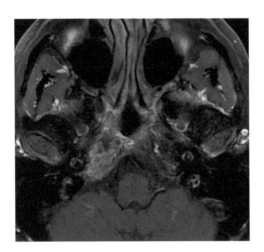

A 45-year-old male presents with right-sided headache.

100.1 What is the **MOST** likely diagnosis?

A. Fibrous dysplasia.

B. Chordoma.

C. Chondrosarcoma.

D. Plasmacytoma.

E. Petrous apicitis.

100.2 Which cranial nerve is **MOST** likely affected in this case?

A. Oculomotor nerve.

B. Trochlear nerve.

C. Trigeminal nerve.

D. Abducens nerve.

E. Facial nerve.

100.3 Which of the following is a characteristic imaging feature of this diagnosis?

A. Midline location.

B. Bony destruction and fragmentation.

C. Restricted diffusion.

D. Intrinsic T1 hyperintensity.

E. Centered on the petrooccipital fissure.

Answers and Explanations

100.1 Correct: C. Chondrosarcoma.

The axial T2-weighted and T1-weighted postcontrast fat-suppressed images show a T2 hyperintense and heterogeneously enhancing mass occurring off midline at the right petrous apex. The characteristic T2 hyperintensity and the off-midline location render chondrosarcoma as the most likely diagnosis.

Other choices and discussion

B. Chordoma is also a notably T2 hyperintense mass; however, this entity is expected to have a midline location.
A, D. Fibrous dysplasia and plasmacytomas are not as T2 hyperintense as chondrosarcomas and chordomas.
E. The presence of a mass-like lesion and relatively mild symptoms exclude petrous apicitis.

100.2 Correct: D. Abducens nerve.

Cranial nerve VI, the abducens nerve, passes over the superior margin of the petrous apex prior to entering the Dorello canal and the cavernous sinus. The extensive petrous apex involvement demonstrated here can result in multiple cranial nerve palsies, with abducens palsy being the most common.

Other choices and discussion

A, C, E. Less commonly involved are oculomotor nerve, trigeminal nerve, and facial nerve.
B. There is no association with trochlear nerve palsy.

100.3 Correct: E. Centered on the petrooccipital fissure.

Chondrosarcoma of the petrous apex is characteristically off-midline and centered on the petrooccipital fissure.

Other choices and discussion

A. In contrast, chordomas are associated with a midline location.
B. Another important distinction is the pattern of bony changes, best seen on CT: chordomas result in bony destruction and fragmentation, whereas chondrosarcomas demonstrate the classic "rings and arcs" chondroid matrix appearance in 50% of the cases.
C, D. In the petrous apex, restricted diffusion is associated with cholesteatoma, and intrinsic T1 hyperintensity is associated with cholesterol granuloma.

References

Chapman PR, Shah R, Curé JK, et al. Petrous Apex Lesions: Pictorial Review. *AJR Am J Roentgenol.* 2011; 196(3 Suppl):WS26–WS37.

Isaacson B, Kutz JW, Roland PS. Lesions of the petrous apex: diagnosis and management. *Otolaryngol Clin North Am.* 2007;40:479–519, viii.

List of Cases   Page